Converting to Phacoemulsification

THIRD EDITION

Making the Transition to In-the-Bag Phaco

Paul S. Koch, MD
Koch Eye Associates
Warwick, Rhode Island

With
Joseph Hoffman
Medical Writer

SLACK Incorporated, 6900 Grove Road, Thorofare, NJ 08086-9447

SLACK International Book Distributors

In Japan:
  Igaku-Shoin, Ltd.
  Tokyo International P.O. Box 5063
  1-28-36 Hongo, Bunkyo-Ku
  Tokyo 113
  Japan

In Canada:
  McGraw-Hill Ryerson Limited
  300 Water Street
  Whitby, Ontario
  L1N 9B6

In all other regions throughout the world, SLACK professional reference books are available through offices and affiliates of McGraw-Hill, Inc. For the name and address of the office serving your area, please correspond to

  McGraw-Hill, Inc.
  Medical Publishing Group
  Attn: International Marketing Director
  1221 Avenue of the Americas — 28th Floor
  New York, NY 10020
  (212)-512-3955 (phone)
  (212)-512-4717 (fax)

Executive Editor: Cheryl D. Willoughby
Publisher: Harry C. Benson

Printed in the United States of America

Library of Congress Catalog Card Number: 91-66240

ISBN: 1-55642-208-3

Published by: SLACK Incorporated
               6900 Grove Road
               Thorofare, NJ 08086-9447

Last digit is print number: 10 9 8 7 6 5 4 3 2 1

To my wife Joanne and my children Katie, age 8, and Paul, age 4, who collectively never cease to encourage me to take on more projects than any sane person should attempt. They suffer because of my work but always with patience, love, and good humor.

Contents

Preface to the Third Edition

Craftsmanship

I had a very good friend come to visit me in surgery recently, and he seemed to enjoy himself quite a bit. He watched carefully everything I did and took a series of notes and about halfway through the day he started asking me questions. They all went something like this: "Paul, I noticed that you did it this way. What's wrong with doing it the old way?" Or, "Paul, I notice that you are not using any stitches. What's wrong with using stitches?"

I patiently explained my opinions and tried to answer his questions as best I could but it dawned on me after awhile that he is suffering from a malady that many of us have to deal with, and I include myself with that many. The malady is inertia. Perhaps it should be called fear. We look around and see other people doing new things, and we suddenly realize that if we do not do the same we will be left behind. I suffer from this disease as well, and when it strikes me it is frightening. Sometimes it is terrifying.

Deep down we know that progress is inevitable. It is impossible to keep performing the old techniques forever. No matter how good we may be at them, it will only be a matter of time before we are a decade or two behind the rest of the world. And in cataract surgery we are already a generation behind if we have not changed our technique within the last three years.

Why is it that some of us work very hard to become better and better cataract surgeons and others do not? No mystery there—it is just a matter of setting one's priorities in life.

About a year ago I gave a talk at the Nassau County College of Surgeons, and part of the talk was spent on discussing how quickly patients can see after sutureless cataract surgery. When the afternoon was over, a very nice ophthalmologist came up to me and asked me point blank why I find it necessary to make patients see so soon after the operation. His patients don't see well for three months, and they don't complain. Why are my patients different that they have to see sooner? Am I not just stirring up a hornet's nest by showing the community that rapid visual rehabilitation is possible?

Frankly, I was a bit taken back by the comments. I had never thought that way before and I tried to explain that rapid recovery after any kind of an operation is better than slow recovery. I was not comfortable with that discussion because I think that his question was driving at something deeper.

It was not until several months had passed that I formulated my thoughts on the subject. I think I could discuss the subject better now given a second chance.

In February 1991 I took my family down to Florida for a vacation. As is my habit, I bought and read a couple of books, which I normally would not have had time for. The first book I read (it has nothing to do with ophthalmology) was Stone Alone. It was written by Bill Wyman, the bass player for the Rolling Stones. I'll give you a little quiz. Do you know who founded the Rolling Stones? No, it was not Mick Jagger and Keith Richards. It was Brian Jones and Ian Stewart. Okay, here is the second half of the quiz. Whatever happened to Ian Stewart? Get ready for this. When the band became popular Ian Stewart was fired because he was considered to be too ugly to be a Rolling Stone. Incredible but true.

Getting closer to the subject at hand, the second book I read was Men at Work by George Will. This is a wonderful book about baseball, in which Will analyzes and dissects all the different people who make up a baseball team: the manager, pitcher, catcher, batter and fielders. In incredible detail, he explains what each individual has to do. The book reads very slowly, almost like a textbook, but over the course of several hundred pages it weaves the indelible notion that baseball is a cerebral activity acted out on a playing field by very talented men. The theme of the book is craftsmanship.

About twenty or thirty pages from the end of the book George Will talks about the movie "Bull Durham." You might have seen this movie. It has to do with minor league baseball and a team, the Durham Bulls, that has a young pitcher who is an incredible talent but very immature. Kevin Costner is an aging catcher brought onto the team to help develop this talented young pitcher. They have a series of squabbles during the course of the film and finally the pitcher turns to Kevin Costner and says, "Why do you hate me so much?" Kevin Costner replies, "I don't hate you, I hate what you think of yourself. Your right arm is worth a million dollars. All the limbs in my body aren't worth seven dollars a pound. But you are content to throw the ball at the plate when you could learn how to pitch the ball to the plate. You are content to throw it as hard as you can when you have the talent to be a very skilled pitcher."

And George Will goes on to explain how this little episode deals with craftsmanship and pride in one's work. He goes on to point out that this applies to many other occupations, and he specifically mentions surgery.

There are people who look on cataract surgery as a craft, who seek to make it better and better every day, who want to become the most perfect cataract surgeons imaginable. There are other people who think that cataract surgery just means slicing an incision into the eye, removing the cataractous lens, replacing it with an implant, and closing the eye up again afterwards. These people could be called journeymen but not craftsmen.

Craftsmanship is the pride one takes in one's work. A craftsman constantly tries to improve his or her craft and become better every day. A surgeon who is not a craftsman will be content with less, and will feel threatened when the craftsmen and craftswomen pull ahead in technique and results.

Fear, paranoia and anger run hand in hand. How many of us have thought to ourselves that we were better than anybody else because we did all the new procedures. Then we turned around and thought that we were better than everybody else because we used all the tried and proved procedures. The psychology of keeping up in medicine is a complicated one.

I am not sure where the anger comes from, but it certainly has been expressed lately. Recently a very good article on astigmatism and small incision surgery ran in the journal Ophthalmology. An accompanying editorial almost apologized for running the article, because the feeling was that many readers would find the subject of astigmatism after cataract surgery trivial. I find it of singular importance, but apparently many others do not.

It is my firm belief that the frictions that occur in ophthalmology and medicine today do not exist between the phacoemulsification surgeons and the extracapsular surgeons. It does not exist between the high volume surgeons and the low volume surgeons. I firmly believe that friction, paranoia, anger and fear exist between the journeymen and the craftsmen.

This book is written for the people who want to be craftsmen and craftswomen. I do not pretend to have all the answers in this book. I pray that by the time it is published much of it will already be out of date, because I hope we are all constantly improving.

I try very hard to be a craftsman, and all the surgeons I respect are definitely craftsmen. I hope that everyone who reads this book will try to be one too.

Preface to the First and Second Editions

This is an intimate book. This is is how I do phacoemulsification and how you might like to do it, too. The techniques, the prejudices, and the editorial directives are all mine.

It's easier to write a ponderous text, quoting some, footnoting others, and referencing many. It's easier, more inclusive, and yet widely exclusive. It's also anonymous.

I've had some good teachers. My first phaco course was with the father, Charles Kelman, MD. The first attending who helped me with phacoemulsification when I was a resident was Peter Berglas, MD. They taught me how to do one-handed anterior chamber phacoemulsification.

The first person I saw do two-handed phacoemulsification was my close friend, Alexander Calenda, MD, who can move two instruments around in the eye as if they were knitting needles. He was years ahead of his time.

I taught myself how to perform posterior chamber phacoemulsification. I spent a week at the Academy watching every phaco tape shown at every booth on the exhibit floor. By the time I went home, I knew I could perform the operation in my sleep.

George Fava, MD, was a classmate of mine in medical school. We were in each other's wedding parties. He understands this operation inside and out, not just knows it, mind you, but really understands it. That's rare. I've picked his brain so many times he must have holes in his head by now.

Sometimes when I get caught up in technology of what we're doing, or frustrated by the politics, or by the economics of modern ophthalmology, I try to keep things in perspective. I'd be doing exactly the same thing even if I had a crystal ball. There's a certain spark that ignites when something is just right. I can feel that spark in the work I do.

My father, Peter Koch, MD, is an anesthesiologist. Thirty years ago he also had a general practice and made house calls. He has that spark. To this day, former patients talk about him. They come to me and hope that I'm something of what they knew him to be. I take a history. They've had three operations. Who was the surgeon? They can't remember, but Dr. Koch gave the anesthesia. Who forgets their surgeon but remembers their anesthesiologist? No one, no time, no place, except here, where they remember my dad. We work together now and he still makes me proud, but I have to dedicate this book to my wife or else she won't talk to me.

It was either the book or the boat, and I already had a name for the boat.

Now light a fire in the fireplace, take your shoes off, relax, and read this book. If you understand what it says, if you can visualize the maneuvers, and if it makes sense to you, I've done my job. If not, it's your problem.

Like I said, this is an intimate book.

Introduction

The third edition of *Converting to Phacoemulsification* is completely rewritten from the first and second editions. Except by some quirk of statistical anomaly there ought not to be a single sentence in common with the first two editions. If you are browsing through this book and you already have one of the earlier editions, please buy this one. My publisher and I will both thank you.

The first and second editions of *Converting to Phacoemulsification* cover iris plane phacoemulsification. It had to do with can opener capsulotomies, running sutures and techniques which are just plain dead as far as many phacoemulsification surgeons are concerned.

This book deals with modern concepts of incisions, with capsulorhexis, with in-the-bag phacoemulsification. This is a completely different world from the previous editions. I used to think that iris plane phacoemulsification was a necessary learning step before proceeding to phacoemulsification in the bag. I no longer think that. I now think that it is possible and, in fact, I believe it is even wise to begin phacoemulsification in the capsular bag. But only when you can picture in your mind how the nucleus functions in the bag. When performing in-the-bag phacoemulsification you have no escape. The decision to perform the operation is the commitment to doing it. Converting is not nearly as easy as it is in iris plane phacoemulsification.

In this book I am going to help you conceptualize what happens inside the eye so you can picture each step and see its role in the greater cosmos of phacoemulsification. All the players should come together and provide a coherent view for what needs to be done in that eye.

We are going to spend a lot of time dealing with topics that were brushed over in the first book. We have a long chapter just dealing with incisions. We have learned that the incision is the most important step of the operation in determining the level of immediate visual rehabilitation.

We are going to define different kinds of cataracts and how the strategy in phacoemulsification has to change depending on what kind of a cataract you are dealing with.

We are going to talk about why the new continuous tear capsulotomies are important. We will talk about the different hydro techniques and what they do.

All in all, a formidable task for a little book. Let's get right to it.

1

Patient Prep and Anesthesia

Pre-medication

We do not use preoperative sedation as a standard part of our patient preparation.

Pupillary dilation

More than any other factor, a larger pupil will make phacoemulsification easier to perform.

Cyclopentolate, tropicamide and phenylephrine are used routinely in our practice, but not flurbiprofen. It is not needed to prevent a miotic response to surgical trauma, which does not typically occur during the relatively short operative time that we usually achieve. Its local anticoagulant effect is also considered a drawback. Flurbiprofen should certainly be considered helpful in the learning stages of phaco, however, where the operation is such that you will have iris irritation and miosis.

Anesthesia and akinesia

You do need an adequate block before every operation. At our facility, I administer the block, then start surgery on a previously prepared patient. The patient who just received the block is checked by the staff. If there is any movement at all, even a twitch of 1 mm, the case is delayed so that the block can be augmented. I would rather give a second injection than the hear a patient say "ouch" when we start to operate.

A two-site, peribulbar-retrobulbar injection method is used, with 3 cc of anesthetic given inferotemporally and 2 cc superonasally. We have found no need to administer a facial block, as this technique has consistently resulted in adequate akinesia as well as anesthesia.

A 5 cc syringe with a 1.5-inch, 25-gauge needle is filled with a mixture of 2% and 4% lidocaine with Wydase. The 4% lidocaine comes in an ampule, and we mix it with 2% lidocaine because it comes in a vial; this enables the Wydase to be combined with the lidocaine and thoroughly mixed by shaking.

We do not use epinephrine, which is potentially painful due to its acidity. (Plain lidocaine has a pH of about 5, but when mixed with epinephrine it is about 3.5!) Neither is Marcaine used, because it can delay the return of useful vision in the immediate postoperative period.

The first injection is made through the lower eyelid just lateral to the inferior rectus muscle. A site about one third of the distance in from the lateral toward the medial canthus is appropriate. The needle is kept vertical as it is inserted, without angling in toward the muscle cone or optic nerve. The needle is passed to a depth of 1 to 1.25 inch. After 3 cc of anesthetic is injected, the patient is instructed to close the eye. The rest of the anesthetic in the syringe is injected just under the superior orbital rim, nasal to the superior rectus muscle. This site is located about one third of the distance from to medial canthus toward the lateral canthus. Gentle massage should confirm that the contents of the orbit are not unusually firm, which would indicate the presence of a hematoma. A Honan balloon is placed for 10 minutes.

Chilled infusion

Chilled infusion solution should certainly be incorporated into this type of phaco surgery. It stabilizes the blood-aqueous barrier, constricts blood vessels and facilitates the transfer of heat away from the phaco probe and out of the eye. With incisions that reach up into the cornea, this last point becomes a very important consideration. In our surgical center, we chill the bottles of saline solution to 4°C, but do not use an ice bath for the infusion tubing as some surgeons recommend. The cooling effect of the chilled solution does not seem to suffer without the ice bath.

2

Incisions

The 1991 ASCRS meeting in Boston was an extraordinary meeting and if you were lucky enough to be sitting in large Auditorium A on Monday then you were fortunate enough to have witnessed a turning point in cataract surgery. That was the day that sutureless cataract surgery was announced to be the new standard of care.

Incisions enter the new decade

The extraordinary thing about this day was that nobody saw it coming. It was only January 1990 that Mike McFarland of Pine Bluffs, Arkansas began teaching people the corneal valve incision. It was not until the summer and the fall of 1990 that people began talking about it and the first few courses popped up teaching the technique. Nothing was written about it. Only a handful of articles appeared in places like Ocular Surgery News and Ophthalmology Times. There was widespread suggestion that this might be a marketing ploy and not an advance in technique and results.

Only three weeks before the ASCRS meeting a fellow was visiting me in surgery and asked me how many people around the country were doing sutureless cataract surgery and I told him I thought there were probably 75 or 100. Imagine my surprise then when I sat in that room on Monday morning and there were 50, 75, maybe even 100 papers on sutureless surgery, and these had been submitted for the meeting way back in November 1990.

When I presented my paper I looked out at the hundreds of people in the auditorium and I could see two kinds of faces. One group was sitting there blissfully smiling because they knew they were on top of things. The rest of the auditorium was sitting there with their jaws touching their knees. It was like they were being hit over the head with a 2 by 4. They came for this meeting as extracapsular surgeons or, even more upsetting, people who had just started doing phaco and thought they were right on top of things. Then they sat down that morning and found out that there were hundreds of people doing something incredibly different with dramatically better results. They had no idea what hit them.

You absolutely must plan to begin performing corneal valve incisions if you are not doing them already. It must be your goal that in six months your routine operation will not require stitches. I will present some statistics later on but for now just believe me—the corneal valve incision (sutureless cataract surgery) is not a gimmick. It is a dramatic breakthrough and one which you must embrace warmly.

Unfortunately, if you do not already perform phacoemulsification a corneal valve incision will make your transition to phaco much more difficult.

What we will do is describe three different types of incision, roughly corresponding to the stages of development of phaco proficiency:

1. The basic incision, emphasizing ease of manipulation of instruments for surgeons who have not done phaco and want to perform it as easily and simply as possible. Once you acquire a familiarity with phaco, you will abandon this incision completely.

2. An intermediate incision, in which you begin to take account of some of the external structural characteristics of the wound that affect the amount of induced astigmatism. This incision introduces the option of horizontal suturing.

3. An advanced self-sealing, corneal valve incision, which is a dramatic improvement over the preceding stages.

If you are not performing phacoemulsification now, I want you to do a basic incision until you get comfortable. Once you are comfortable with phacoemulsification (or if you are already) I want you to jump right on ahead to the intermediate incision. As soon as you are comfortable there, I want you to abandon that and go right to the corneal valve incision, and then stay there until we invent something new.

Technique

The basic incision: For early transition period

The basic incision maximizes your ability to maneuver the instruments inside the eye. It does not give you a lot of control over astigmatism, but that is not the goal of this incision. At this point, we want to make an incision that will make learning phaco easier. Astigmatism considerations will come later.

Two components. The basic incision consists of two components, an external incision and an internal incision. The external incision is the groove that you place in the sclera and the internal incision is your entry into the anterior chamber.

The closer you are to the limbus, the more maneuverability your phaco tip will have. If you have a long tunnel of tissue compressing the top of the tip, it will have very little maneuverability. If you have only a thin bridge of tissue sitting on top of your phaco tip, you will be able to move that tip like an oar in an oarlock. For this reason the basic incision is a very anterior incision.

When making a basic incision, a groove in the sclera (the external incision) should be placed in white tissue just far enough back so that there is enough white tissue for the anterior placement of your suture bites (Figure 2-1). You do not want to put sutures in clear cornea or in blue tissue. As long as you leave a little bit of white tissue in which to pass the stitch, you are far enough back. For the more quantitative minded, you are 0.5 to 1 mm off the cornea into white tissue.

Anterior chamber entry. Depending on the exact placement of the external incision, you might find it necessary to dissect up a little flap toward the limbus or you might not need to. Sometimes you can take your blade and stab from the bottom of that groove directly into the anterior chamber (Figure 2-2). As far as I am concerned, when you are using the basic incision either approach is fine.

However you may choose to reach the anterior chamber, the internal incision must be off the iris. There has to be a lip between the internal entry point and the iris. This is important for several reasons. The main one is that it physically separates your phaco tip from the iris. This makes it less likely that iris will wash out of the incision and less likely that you will rub the phaco tip on the iris. Rubbing the phaco tip on the iris irritates it and causes miosis. That will just make the operation more difficult. Furthermore, the tissue damage from rubbing the iris can release prostaglandins, possibly

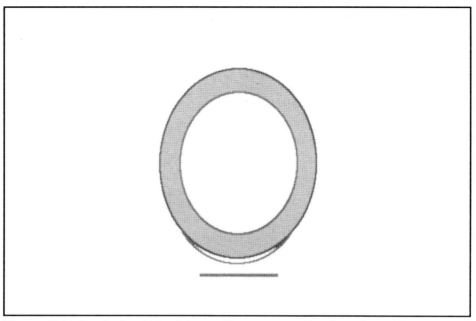

Figure 2-1. In the basic incision, a linear groove in the sclera (the external incision) should be placed just far enough back from the limbus so that there is enough white tissue for placement of suture bites.

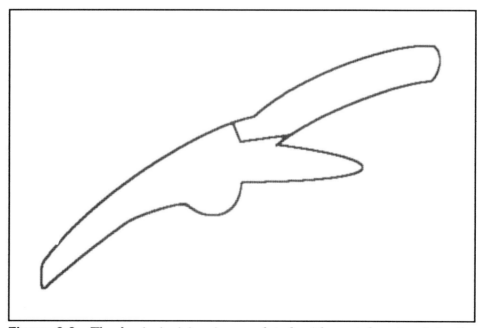

Figure 2-2. The basic incision is completed with a stab entry into the anterior chamber. Depending on the exact placement of the external incision, it will occasionally be necessary to dissect a flap up toward the limbus.

causing cystoid macular edema. A little bit of separation is all you need to prevent some of these untoward side effects.

If you enter the eye and you find that you are right on top of the iris, do not despair. You can pull the blade back again, aim it a little more anterior, and stab it into the eye a second time. From then on, as long as you use only the second incision, the first, more posterior incision will be compressed and sealed throughout the operation. It will cause you no difficulty.

When you enter the anterior chamber you should plan to use a keratome of approximately 3.0 mm in width. The exact width of your keratome would depend on the phacoemulsification machine that you use. We had previously taught that you first should enter the eye with a small blade for the capsulotomy but now we are almost universally using forceps for the continuous tear capsulotomy, so we need a bigger opening.

Side-Port Incision. Another incision is placed 90° away in clear cornea at approximately two o'clock. A narrow keratome or a pointed blade can be used to make this incision parallel to the iris, approximately 1.5 mm inside clear cornea. This is where we will introduce the spatula in our two-handed phaco technique. This incision is always self-sealing, provided it is not made too large or perpendicular to the surface of the cornea.

Do not neglect this second incision. Not only is it useful during the operation as a place to put your spatula and inject viscoelastic, but it is also useful on the day after surgery. If the patient has high pressure in the eye the next day, it is a very simple matter to press on that side port incision at the slit lamp with any sort of sterile instrument and let some aqueous leak out of the eye. It is possible to reduce an intraocular pressure from 60 to 6 mm Hg in a matter of a second or two. I firmly believe that even if you are performing one-handed phacoemulsification (a technique that I do not recommend) you ought to make the side port incision anyway because it gives you access to the eye and leaves a pressure valve for the day after surgery.

That is about it for the basic incision. It is very simple, it is fairly anterior and it maximizes maneuverability. It is not a sophisticated incision but it is not meant to be. I think it is the best incision to use when you are learning phacoemulsification because it makes the operation easier. I do not think it is a good incision when held up against the next two we'll be looking at.

The intermediate incision: A scleral pocket technique

The intermediate incision is what is usually called the scleral pocket incision. The scleral pocket was described about ten years ago by Richard Kratz, and it remains one of the best ways to have a small, stable, secure incision when performing phacoemulsification. About two years ago there was a big trend toward combining the scleral pocket incision with horizontal suturing techniques. This was a breakthrough and remains my technique of choice when I have to use a suture. Here is how the scleral pocket incision is made.

For this incision we move the vertical groove a little more posterior on the sclera until we are 1 or even 2 mm behind the blue zone of the limbus (Figure 2-3). The length of the groove is directly related to the diameter of the intraocular lens that is going to be used. For purposes of this discussion we will call it 6 mm long. After the vertical groove is made, a scleral tunnel is dissected from the groove toward the anterior chamber (Figure 2-4). The tunnel should be mid-thickness in the sclera.

The dissection can be made with one of a number of instruments. A diamond knife can be used, a metal scleral dissecting blade can be used, and even the sides of a keratome can be used. The idea is to

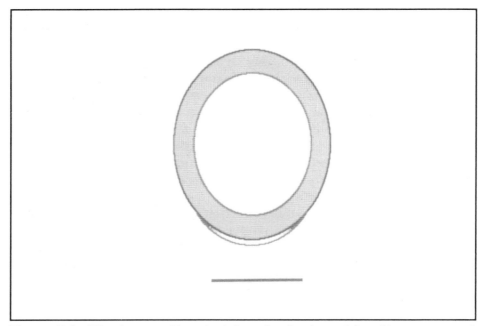

Figure 2-3. The intermediate incision also begins with a linear external incision, but it is made further back from the limbus than in the basic incision.

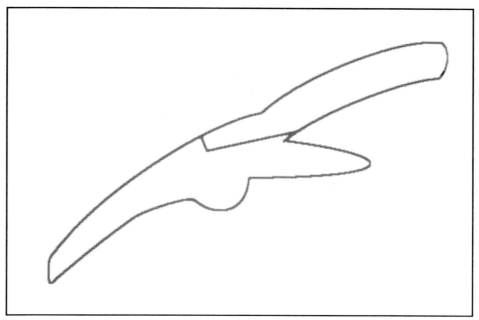

Figure 2-4. A scleral tunnel is then dissected from the groove up to the anterior chamber.

make a uniplanar connection of the scleral groove to the anterior chamber. When the groove dissection reaches the anterior chamber, the chamber is entered with the keratome corresponding to the phaco tip width.

There is really only one problem with the scleral pocket incision: some limitation of mobility of the instruments. But this is a small problem and, except for the beginner, I do not think it should interfere with our decision to use this incision. Another minor disadvantage has to do with lens insertion. When you push the intraocular lens through the tunnel there is a point where the optic is trapped and, if the lens has anteriorly angled haptics, they can approach the corneal endothelium. Again, I think that is a small matter and one that is easily controlled with firm application of instrumentation during lens insertion.

Some people complain about the incidence of hyphemas after a scleral pocket incision. This is a subject which we will dismiss now and discuss in some detail in the next section. There may be an increased incidence of hyphemas if you use a running stitch at the scleral groove, but there is no increased risk if you use a horizontal stitch or modify the scleral tunnel into a corneal valve incision.

There are a bunch of advantages to using this intermediate incision instead of the basic incision. The main one is that it leads to

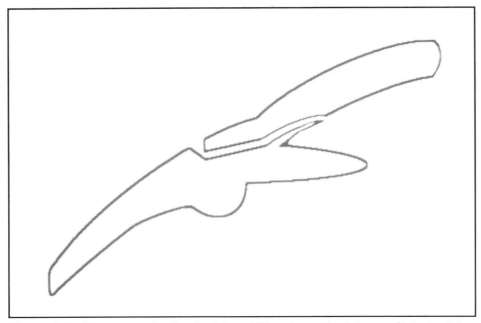

Figure 2-5. The corneal valve incision differs from the intermediate incision in the anterior chamber entry. The tunnel dissection is carried up into the corneal stroma before the stab entry into the chamber is made.

a more secure wound and because the incision is further back from the limbus there is less stimulus for the production of astigmatism. Once again, this is a topic which we will discuss in the next section. For purposes of this discussion, it suffices to say that the scleral pocket is better than the basic incision at limiting the induction of astigmatism and assuring postoperative astigmatism stability.

The corneal valve incision for sutureless surgery

Now comes the good stuff. The corneal valve incision is almost exactly the same thing as the scleral pocket incision, except that when you dissect your pocket up toward the anterior chamber you spend a little more time in the cornea. When you dissect up toward the anterior chamber and you reach the cornea, dissect a little more anterior within the corneal stroma before entering the eye (Figure 2-5). This entry point is the astigmatism control point (as we will discuss in moment).

The dissection into clear cornea means that you are constructing a corneal valve. That's it, that's the entire thing.

The corneal tissue is soft, flexible and compressible. That means the dissection into clear cornea can be squeezed tight by pressure

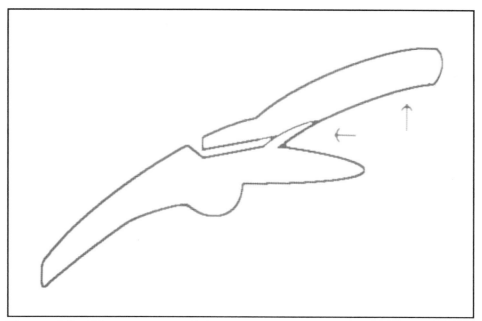

Figure 2-6. The incision will be closed by normal intraocular pressure against the flexible corneal tissue.

against the endothelium from within the anterior chamber (Figure 2-6). It is the pressure in the eye that closes the incision. The more pressure in the eye, the stronger the incision.

Now might be a good time to introduce some structural considerations and statistics to show how changing the incision even a little bit can lead to dramatically better results.

Discussion

Structural principles

The incision is more than a port of access to the anterior segment, as it is the most important step of the operation insofar as ocular integrity and corneal stability are concerned.

As you recall, there are actually two incisions that need to be considered: the external incision and the internal incision. The external incision is both the groove on the sclera and the tunnel up to the anterior chamber. The internal incision is the actual entry into the eye. Both of them must work in harmony in order for the incision to serve its full function as an entry port and as the focus for corneal stability.

Let us consider first some common external incisions. A very common and traditional incision is a curvilinear one following the curve of the limbus (Figure 2-7A). There is nothing about this incision to prevent the inferior edge from falling away from the superior edge (Figure 2-7B). This wound gape potential is the cause of against-the-rule astigmatism.

If the curvilinear incision is changed to a straight incision (Figure 2-8A), a few things happen. The two extreme points of the incision are secured in the sclera, and the inferior edge of the incision directly adjacent to these end points of the incision cannot sag (Figure 2-8B). The edges cannot sag, so induced astigmatism is limited to the degree of instability of the middle of the incision. The potential for against-the-rule astigmatism is lessened with this incision, compared to the curvilinear incision, by the simple modification of placing the sides more superiorly on the sclera.

Frown and chevron incisions

If the ends of the incision are placed further superior on the sclera, we have an even more stable incision. Jack Singer's frown incision aims for that goal. The frown differs from previous incisions in that the ends are swept superiorly, away from the limbus (Figure 2-9).

Now things are dramatically different. It is almost as though there are slings hanging down which are supporting the ends of the incision. It is difficult to imagine how the inferior edge of the incision could sag away from the superior edge of the incision. The potential for against-the-rule astigmatism is reduced to virtually nothing.

Another interesting incision along these lines is Sam Pallin's chevron. It is much like the frown, except that it is made with two

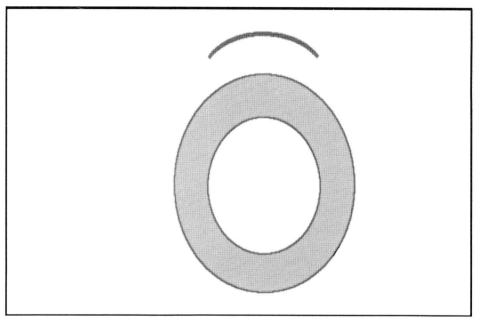

Figure 2-7A. Curvilinear incisions following the curve of the limbus are very commonly used.

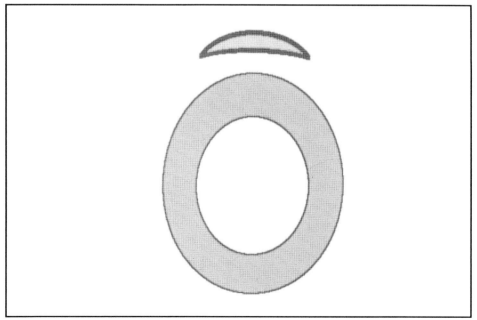

Figure 2-7B. These incisions have a tendency to gape since there is no structural support for the inferior edge of the incision.

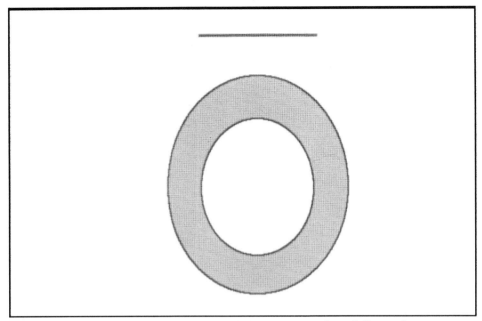

Figure 2-8A. Straight-line incisions behave somewhat differently.

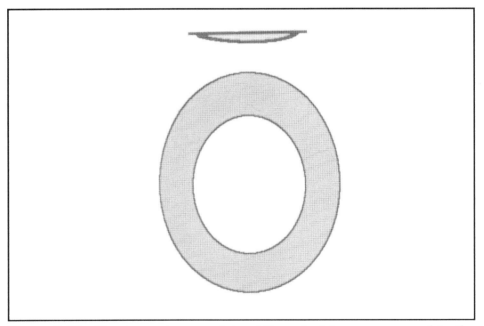

Figure 2-8B. The two extreme points of these incisions are secured in the sclera, so the inferior edge has less tendency to separate from the superior edge.

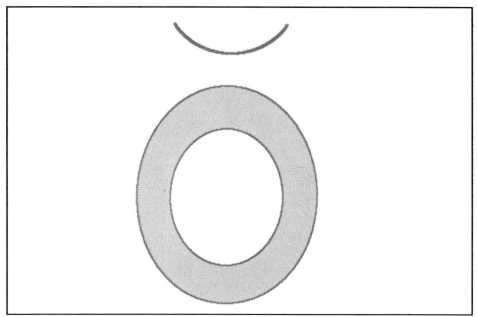

Figure 2-9. The frown incision developed by Jack Singer places the ends of the incision far superiorly to better support the inferior edge.

straight cuts rather than one curved cut. In both techniques, the sides of the incision sweep away from the cornea. Jack Singer likes to describe the stability of these incisions as being like the center span on a suspension bridge, but that's only part of the story.

The incisional funnel

The relationship between the shape of the external incision and astigmatism can be considered in light of a couple of mathematical relationships concerning incision length and corneal astigmatism. Doug Koch performed studies on cadaver eyes to evaluate incision length and astigmatism. Jim Gills analyzed Koch's work and concluded that corneal astigmatism is directly proportional to the cube of the length of the incision (Figure 2-10A,B).

If we also consider that astigmatism is inversely proportional to the distance the incision is placed from the limbus, we can derive a more complete understanding of the mechanics of the external incision. Through a composite description of the interactions among astigmatism, length of incision and distance from the limbus, we arrive at a relationship I call the incisional funnel.

The incisional funnel is bounded by a pair of curved lines whose shape is based on the relationship between astigmatism and two

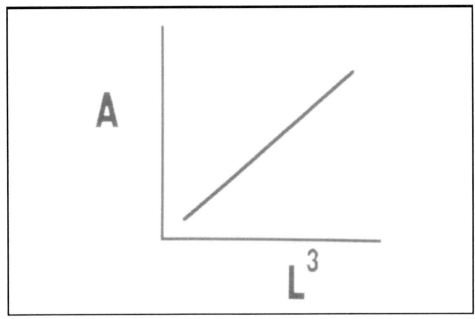

Figure 2-10A. Jim Gills' analysis of Doug Koch's study of incision length versus astigmatism determined that induced astigmatism (A) is proportional to the cube of the incision length (L).

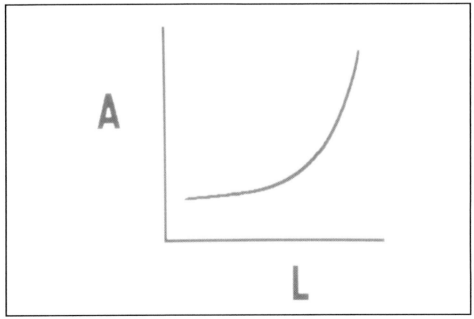

Figure 2-10B. The graph of A versus L (not cubed) shows how astigmatism increases rapidly as the incision increases in length.

characteristics of incisions: incision length and the distance from the limbus. Incisions made within this funnel will be, for all practical purposes, astigmatism equivalent. Short incisions can be made closer to the limbus and longer ones further away, and all will have equivalent corneal stability (Figure 2-11A-F).

A curvilinear incision made parallel to the limbus falls out of the incisional funnel and is unstable. The straight incision placed at the same distance still falls outside the funnel, but not as much. It is more stable than the curvilinear incision but not as stable as the frown or chevron incisions, which lie entirely within the funnel.

Moving the linear incision further away from the limbus will make it more stable. Unfortunately, a more posterior placement of the incision also hampers surgery by increasing the length of the tunnel and restricting the movement of the instruments. These restrictions are less bothersome when a frown or chevron incision is made, because while the chord length of the external incision remains the same, the middle of the incisions are closer to the limbus, shortening the tunnel distance and freeing up instrument movement.

The incisional gape

When an incision is made on the scleral surface it is common to see the two edges of the incision separate from each other. This separation, the incisional gape, is a normal, physiologic reaction to two factors: the natural elasticity of the sclera and scleral shrinkage from cautery (Figure 2-12).

The incisional gape does not affect corneal astigmatism. Think about it. If a scleral incision were made and an incisional gape resulted, but then the operation were halted, there would be no net effect on astigmatism (Figure 2-12A,B). The incisional gape in itself is astigmatism neutral.

If we were to continue the incision, tunnelling a flap up to the cornea, but again stopped the case without entering the anterior chamber, there would be still no net effect on the astigmatism (Figure 2-12C). The scleral tunnel is also astigmatism neutral.

Only if we continue the incision and enter the anterior chamber can we have changes in corneal astigmatism. The through-and-through entry into the anterior chamber permits the cornea to change shape (Figure 2-12D). We need to consider, then, that the part of the incision which leads to corneal instability is the entry site, not the external groove and tunnel.

This would explain why we have such little luck controlling astigmatism back at the external incision. Changes in wound placement, suture density and suture tightness have not been able to

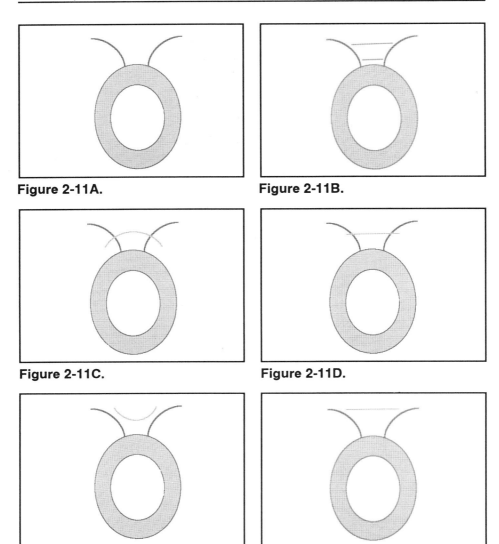

Figure 2-11A.

Figure 2-11B.

Figure 2-11C.

Figure 2-11D.

Figure 2-11E.

Figure 2-11F.

Figure 2-11. A. The incisional funnel is bounded by a pair of lines whose shape is based upon the relationship between astigmatism and two characteristics of incisions: length and the distance from the limbus. Incisions made within this funnel will be astigmatism equivalent. **B.** Short linear incisions made close to the limbus and longer ones further away will have equivalent corneal stability. **C.** A curvilinear incision made parallel to the limbus crosses out of the incisional funnel and is unstable. **D.** The straight incision placed at the same distance still falls outside the funnel, but not by as much. It is more stable than the curvilinear incision but not as stable as the frown or chevron incisions (**E**) which lie entirely within the funnel. **F.** Moving the linear incision further away from the limbus will make it more stable, but also hampers surgery by increasing the length of the tunnel and restricting the movement of the instruments.

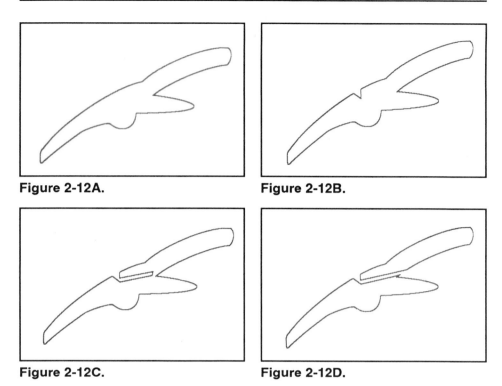

Figure 2-12A. **Figure 2-12B.**

Figure 2-12C. **Figure 2-12D.**

Figure 2-12. Incisional gape, an external phenomenon, is unrelated to induced postoperative corneal astigmatism. **A.** The incision site is structurally sound preoperatively. **B.** If the external scleral groove were to be made and the operation aborted, there would be a wound gape but the structure of the tissues remains essentially intact. There would be no net astigmatic change possible. **C.** Continuing the operation by making a scleral tunnel, then aborting the procedure, would still be astigmatism neutral. **D.** Only after the anterior chamber is entered, violating the structural integrity of the incision site, does corneal instability occur and induce astigmatism.

control astigmatism because the external incision is not the site of corneal instability. In fact, much of what we do at the external incision during closure disturbs the astigmatism control site and actually causes astigmatism.

True effects of suture methods

Radial sutures, for example, are generally placed to approximate the edges of the incision. However, prior to entering the eye, prior to changing corneal stability, the edges were not approximated. They were separated by the normal, physiologic incisional gape. Approximating the edges of the external incision pulls the scleral flap and cornea to a new, unphysiologic position and separates and disturbs the internal entry site, the true astigmatism control site (Figure 2-13). Radial sutures are part of the cause of, not the solution to, corneal astigmatism.

Horizontal sutures, on the other hand, do not attempt to approximate the edges of the incision. They are used simply to flatten the scleral tunnel and make the incision watertight (Figure 2-14). Elimination of the vertical vectors leads to a more physiologic incision closure. Horizontal sutures are less likely to disturb the alignment of the internal entry incision, and that is why they are less likely to cause astigmatism than radial sutures.

But still the closure is made in the scleral tunnel, and the scleral tunnel by itself is astigmatism neutral. A better incision closure would be one that closes the incision close to the internal entry site. Closing the wound where corneal instability and astigmatism are triggered makes the postsurgical wound as physiologic and as stable as possible. This is the natural conclusion of the corneal valve incision

When the intraocular pressure builds up in an eye with a traditional incision, aqueous leaks out unless the incision is secured with sutures (Figure 2-15). When the pressure builds up in the eye

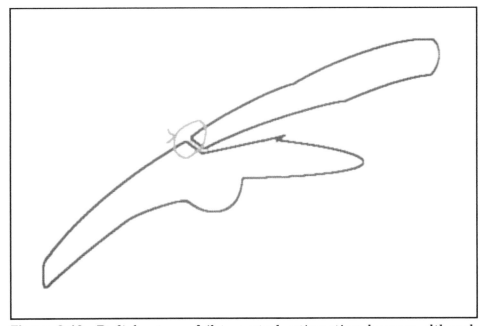

Figure 2-13. Radial sutures fail to control astigmatism because although they reapproximate the edges of the external incision, the scleral flap and cornea are pulled to a new, unphysiologic position and the anterior chamber entry site is disturbed.

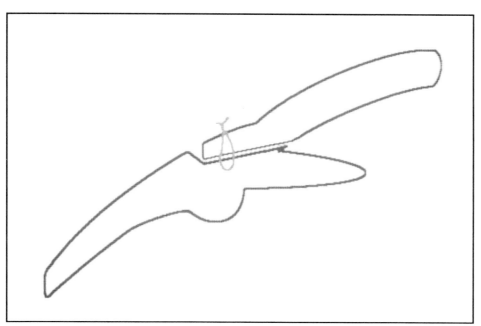

Figure 2-14. Horizontal sutures flatten the scleral tunnel, allowing the external incision to gape but creating a more physiologic closure of the tunnel and internal incision.

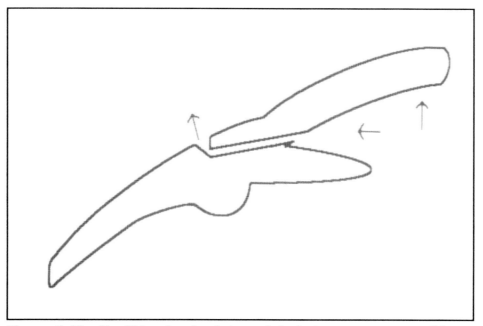

Figure 2-15. Traditional scleral tunnel techniques are susceptible to aqueous leak. Pressure in the anterior chamber pushes up on the cornea, tending to open the tunnel and allow fluid to leak out the eye (arrows). These incisions must be sutured to prevent aqueous loss.

with a corneal valve incision, it presses against the intracorneal portion of the incision, sealing the corneal valve and making the incision watertight without sutures. As the pressure increases, the corneal valve incision becomes tighter.

Koch study of incision size and closure

At the 1991 ASCRS meeting I presented data on astigmatism and visual acuity in a series of almost 700 cases with one of four types of wound closure: 6-mm incision with a running suture; 5-mm incision with a running suture; 5-mm incision with a horizontal suture; and a 5-mm self-sealing corneal valve incision. Induced astigmatism was measured in all patients with at least 6 months of follow up (Figure 2-16).

With a 6-mm incision and a running suture, we found an average of about 1.5 D of induced astigmatism (Table 2-1). Changing to a 5-mm incision while keeping the rest of the technique the same (including the running suture), we saw the average drop to

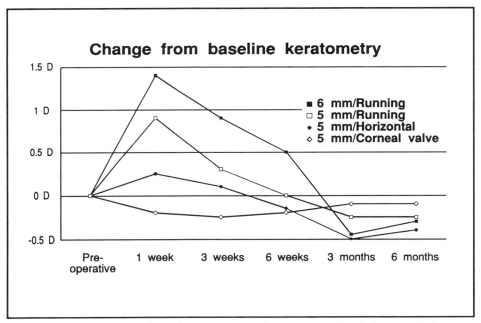

Figure 2-16. Results of study comparing four types of incisions and closure: 6-mm incision with a running suture; 5-mm incision with a running suture; 5-mm incision with a horizontal suture; and a 5-mm self-sealing corneal valve incision. Induced astigmatism was measured in all patients with at least 6 months of follow up.

Incision size and closure method	Number of patients	Average induced astigmatism
6 mm/Running	98	1.5 D
5 mm/Running	73	0.88 D
5 mm/Horizontal	279	0.3 D
5 mm /Corneal valve	239	0.24 D
Total patients studied	689	

Table 2-1. Induced astigmatism for four groups with various incision sizes and closure methods.

about 0.88 D. We then changed the suture method to a horizontal stitch, again changing nothing else about the operation, and the average induced astigmatism dropped to about 0.3 D. With the corneal valve, the average was 0.24 D.

We also examined uncorrected visual acuity. (Best-corrected visual acuity data hide a multitude of sins.) The best uncorrected visual acuity (Figure 2-17) corresponded highly with the type of closure. The 6-mm running stitch group had the worst and the 5-mm corneal valve incision group had the best uncorrected acuities.

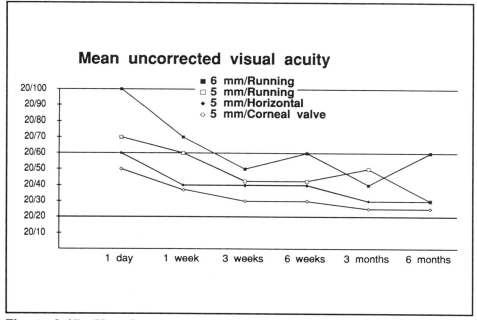

Figure 2-17. Visual acuity measurements in study of incision size and closure method.

Protective functions of valve flap

Corneal tissue's flexibility helps make the corneal valve incision self-sealing. When normal intraocular pressure returns to the postoperative eye, the cornea is pushed back into place and the valve closes. This is the primary function of the incision design.

The shelf left between the plane of entry and the iris also prevents iris prolapse and chafing of the iris by the surgical instruments. Iris chafing leads to miosis, and nothing is less desirable during phaco. The release of prostaglandins, chemical triggers of cystoid macular edema, also results from iris chafing.

The iris in phaco is almost a different tissue from the iris in nucleus expression surgery. Cortical I&A after ECCE is not going to show you what phaco is like. When you use an automated technique of cortex removal after nucleus expression, there will not be any trouble working around the iris. With the cataract gone, the iris is concave and falls away from the incision. In phaco, the cataract is in place and the iris is convex. You have trouble entering the eye with the instruments because the iris is bowed up toward the dome of the cornea. When fluid starts circulating in the anterior chamber it can get between the cataract and the iris, lifting it even higher and forcing it out the incision. If that happens, the iris can lose its structure and become a floppy, depigmented, unmanageable tissue.

Safety of corneal valve

Paul Ernest did an experiment that he presented at the 1991 ASCRS meeting as a videotape. In this experiment, he tested the safety of various sizes and types of incision and closure in eye bank eyes. Fluid infusion was used to build up pressure in the anterior chamber until the wound failed. Standard 8-mm ECCE surgery with interrupted sutures held to about 300 mm Hg before the wound ruptured. With smaller wounds and with scleral incisions further back from the limbus, higher pressures (about 400 mm Hg) were attained before the wounds failed. There were even some eyes obtained with healed cataract incisions. These wounds also ruptured under pressure of around 400 mm Hg. With corneal valve incisions, however, the entire range of pressure measurable on the equipment—from 8 to over 2,000 mm Hg—could be applied without a single unsutured wound leaking.

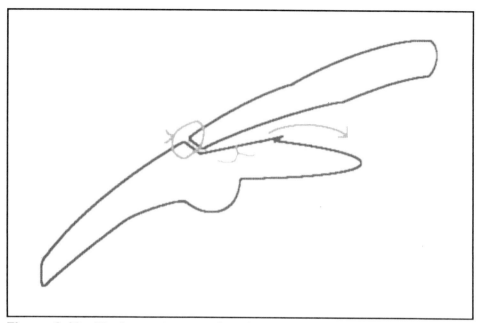

Figure 2-18. Hyphema is exacerbated by radial closure methods, which pinch off the external incision and force blood from the vascular part of the sclera back into the anterior chamber.

Hyphema

Incision construction and closure also affect the rate of postoperative hyphema formation. Let us consider a representative incision which has a bleeding vessel in the floor of the tunnel.

If we close the incision by placing sutures at the edge of the incision, we trap the blood in the tunnel and the only direction it can flow is into the eye (Figure 2-18).

If we place a horizontal suture to flatten the tunnel, one of three things can happen: the suture can tamponade the vessel and bleeding will stop; if the suture is closer to the incision than the bleeding vessel, blood will be directed into the anterior chamber (Figure 2-19A); and if the suture is closer to the anterior chamber than the bleeding vessel, blood will be directed out of the eye through the external incision (Figure 2-19B).

If we have a corneal valve incision, blood cannot flow into the anterior chamber because the closure is between the bleeding point and the anterior chamber. As a result, all of the blood must flow out

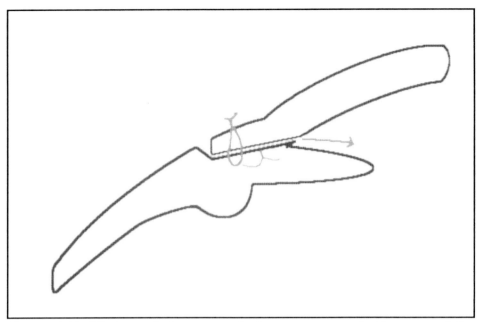

Figure 2-19. Horizontal closure methods can tamponade the area of the vessels, stopping the bleeding, or may have one of two other effects.

A. If the suture is closer to the incision than the bleeding vessel, blood will be directed into the anterior chamber.

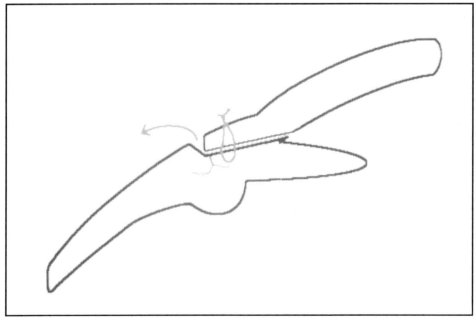

Figure 2-19B. If the suture is closer to the anterior chamber than the bleeding vessel, blood will be directed out of the eye through the external incision.

through the external incision (Figure 2-20).

Data from our study of incisions bear out these conclusions (Table 2-2).

Scleral disinsertion

There are reports of patients with several diopters of against-the-rule astigmatism in cases in which a tunnel incision was closed with a single horizontal stitch, or in cases in which a corneal valve incision

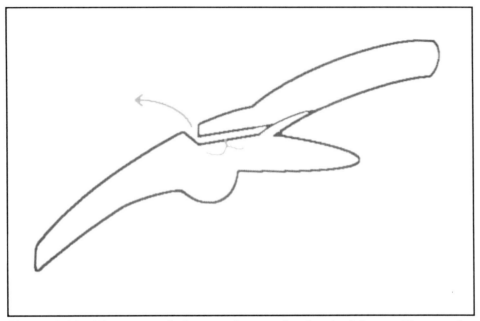

Figure 2-20. The internal closure of corneal valve incisions will never let blood flow into the anterior chamber, but instead will always force it out through the external incision.

Eyes	Suture	# Hyphema	Hyphema
320	Running	22	7
500	Horizontal	20	4
300	Corneal Valve	1	0.3

Table 2-2. Incidence of hyphema in study of incision size and closure methods based on type of closure used.

was used. Gerry Spindel reviewed several of these cases and noticed that in each case, the initial groove incision was very deep, in some cases right down to the supraciliary space. In each case he found more than average incisional gaping.

A very deep groove incision can cause scleral disinsertion: the complete separation of the inferior sclera from the sclera superior to the incision. Unless there is a bridge of tissue (Figure 2-21), there is no support for the sclera from the groove to the limbus. Incision closure on the inferior side of the incision, whether by means of a horizontal stitch or corneal valve, is unable to provide any support.

In cases of scleral disinsertion, it will be necessary to use radial or horizontal mattress sutures to secure the edges of the incision on either side of the scleral groove (Figure 2-22). Prevention of scleral disinsertion is by making the groove incision only partial thickness, either by judicious use of a freehand incision or with a guarded blade designed for this purpose.

Conclusion

The incision is not just a port of access to the anterior chamber, it is the most important structural variable in cataract surgery. Under-

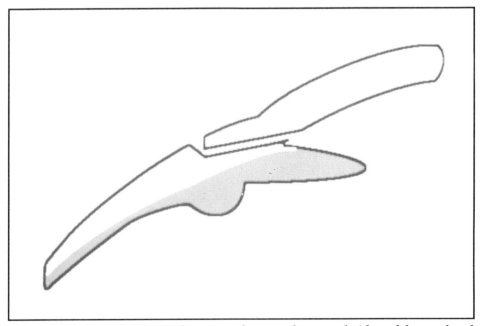

Figure 2-21. A properly made external groove leaves a bridge of deep scleral tissue (gray area) from one side of the incision to the other.

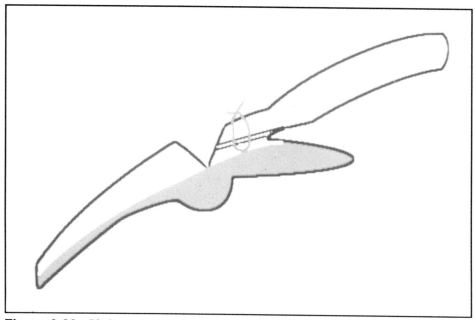

Figure 2-22. If the groove is too deep, scleral disinsertion results. Without the bridge of deep scleral tissue, there is no support for the sclera from the groove to the limbus. It will be necessary to use radial or horizontal mattress sutures to secure the edges of the incision on either side of the scleral groove.

stand the implications of the structural changes, and you understand how to make more secure and stable incisions.

The principles of the external and internal incisions also help us to focus on the entry site as a more specific location for the site of corneal instability.

Further analysis will define the limits of astigmatism-free surgery, the point at which incision size ceases to play a role in astigmatism, and the maximum tolerances consistent with astigmatism-free surgery.

Making the Transition

In converting from extracapsular cataract extraction (ECCE) to phacoemulsification, you will be changing your incision in a series of stages. Even before you have a phaco unit in the operating room, you can practice making the corneal valve incision as described above.

The typical incision for nucleus expression is made just behind the limbus and extends for about 100° around the eye. To begin the transition to the basic phaco incision, try to shift your incision away from the limbus. Move it back a little further in each subsequent case and do a tunnel dissection. You can practice by making the 4- to 6-mm phaco incision, then extending it to the width necessary to perform your standard nucleus expression technique.

Scissors are not used to enlarge the incision. The same blade used to make the initial incision should be used so that the plane established within the sclera can be maintained. In this way, the work done in practicing for phaco will improve the results of your extracaps. You will have a stronger wound and less induced astigmatism, even when this type of incision is used with a nucleus expression technique.

3

Anterior Capsulotomy

The continuous tear capsulotomy, also called capsulorhexis or continuous curvilinear capsulotomy (CCC), is the single biggest breakthrough in cataract surgery of the past ten years—flat out, no beating around the bush. The continuous tear capsulotomy is what made it possible for us to move to in-the-bag phacoemulsification. It made possible all of the new techniques and challenged us to find new and better ways to remove cataracts to take advantage of its unique qualities.

That said, let's admit that capsulorhexis can be one of the hardest techniques to learn. Although some surgeons take to capsulorhexis immediately, you might need a few dozen cases before you enjoy doing it. For starters, don't bother with a bent-needle capsulorhexis. It's slower and harder to learn than what we'll be doing.

Technique

Circular continuous tear capsulotomy

There are a lot of people who perform this capsulotomy with a needle and a lot who do it with the forceps. I think the forceps technique is dramatically easier than the needle technique and I think this is what you ought to learn.

Begin the capsulotomy by using a blunt cystitome to raise a small Christmas tree flap (Figure 3-1). This technique was popularized by Charles Kelman twenty years ago. It has fallen out of favor because people have been doing can opener capsulotomies, but it is a technique that needs to be resurrected.

I am really talking about a number of different instruments when I refer to a blunt cystitome. The most common one is simply a reusable Kelman blunt cystitome. It's just like the sharp one, except that it has a dull tip. There is also a Kelman double cystitome with two dull prongs on the end that help make the flap. A disposable cystitome designed by Bob Kellan is shaped something like a pointed hoe, and it virtually always gives a nice flap.

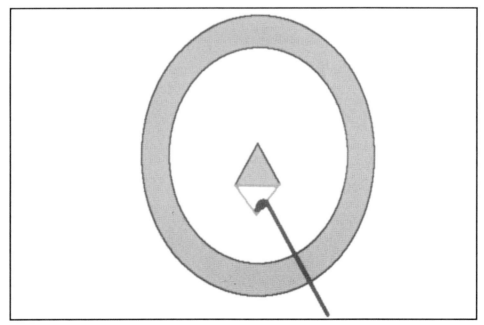

Figure 3-1. The continuous tear anterior capsulotomy is begun by pulling the capsule toward the incision with a blunt cystitome. This raises a small Christmas tree flap.

Gently engage the anterior capsule with the blunt cystitome. Rather than cutting it, you can pull on the middle of the anterior capsule and tease it toward the incision. When you do this, the capsule will tear in a triangular fashion, raising a flap. You can then grab this flap with a pair of capsulotomy forceps to make the continuous tear. I do not think it matters which capsulotomy forceps you use. They are all patterned after the wonderful design of Peter Utrata: long-angled forceps with two points at the tip directed downward to grasp the anterior capsule. They all work well.

For purposes of this discussion we will make the circular tear in a counterclockwise fashion.

Grasp the triangular flap at the corner, pointing toward the 1 o'clock position (Figure 3-2). (As you stare at the eye that will be the corner of the flap in the lower left hand portion of your microscope image.) Grab the flap right near the end of the cut, pull it gently toward 12 o'clock and then quickly around toward 7 o'clock. When you do this the tear will come toward you, then turn and head away from you. As soon as the tear begins to go away from you, stop pulling. Go back and regrasp the base of the anterior capsule flap. It is critically important that you stop the tear at least every three clock hours and

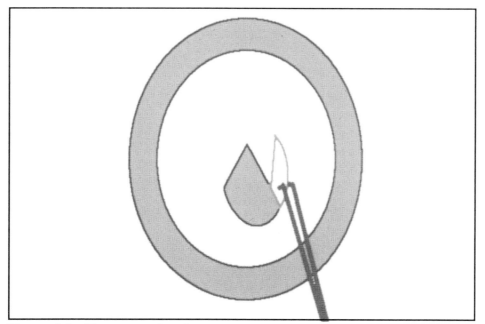

Figure 3-2. The triangular flap is grasped near its base with capsulorhexis forceps. The tear is continued by pulling the flap gently toward 12 o'clock and then quickly around toward 7 o'clock. This will bring the tear toward you, then it will turn and head away.

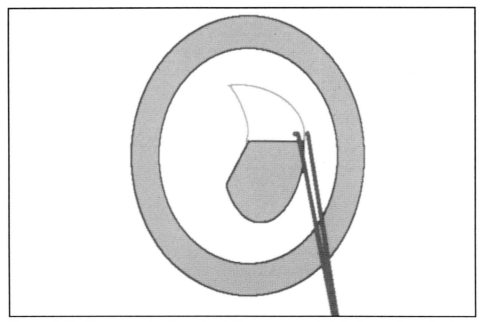

Figure 3-3. The capsular flap should be regrasped at its base when the tear starts heading away from you. It is important to regrasp the base of the flap every three clock hours to maintain control.

regrasp the anterior capsule near the point where the continuous tear terminates. Stop more often and regrasp if that works better for you.

You will soon get a feel for watching how the anterior capsule tears. You will find that the tear proceeds in a circle outside the circle made by your forceps. In other words, the forceps move in a circle with a smaller radius than the circular tear.

Back to our tear-in-progress. Tear the capsule until it reaches the 9 o'clock position. Stop, let go, and regrasp the capsule at its base right next to the termination of the tear and make a second movement to tear the flap down toward 6 o'clock (Figure 3-3). Stop, regrasp and tear the capsule by pulling it toward 9 o'clock. Stop, regrasp again and tear toward 12 o'clock.

As the tear reaches the 12 o'clock position and approaches the starting point, guide the tear so that it is outside the original one and then bring your forceps down toward the 7 o'clock position. This will finish the tear from the outside in, and a smooth capsulotomy will be completed (Figure 3-4).

Try to aim for an anterior capsulotomy of about 5 mm in diameter. It is possible to make them 6 or even 7 mm in diameter, but it is difficult and, because the edge is so close to the pupil and likely to disappear around the equator, large capsulorhexes are much more difficult to control. It is very easy to make a capsulotomy 3 or 4 mm in diameter, but it is very hard to work through them.

Kellan's pear-shaped capsulotomy

I have a very good friend by the name of Bob Kellan who has a very practical approach to life. When he sees something that seems difficult, he tries to find ways to make it simple. I love the way he thinks. Bob noticed how difficult some people found the continuous tear capsulotomy, made a few observations and devised a rather unusual shape for his capsulorhexis.

His first observation was that the important thing about capsulorhexis was its continuous tear, not its shape. Capsulotomies of different sizes, shapes and orientations all seemed to have the same equivalent effect. The key was the preservation of the nearly intact capsular bag. Mild asymmetries in the anterior capsulotomy do not seem to lead to significant asymmetries in intraocular lens placement.

The next observation Bob made was that the difficult part of the capsulotomy was when he had to push away from the incision with

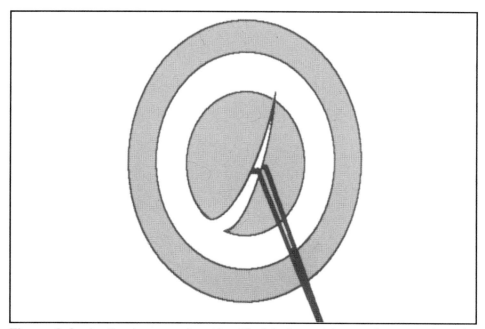

Figure 3-4. As the tear reaches the 12 o'clock position and approaches the starting point, the tear is guided outside the original turning point and the forceps are brought down toward the 7 o'clock position. This will finish the tear from the outside in, and a smooth capsulotomy will be completed.

the forceps. Pulling toward the incision was a much more natural motion, so he wondered if it possible to create a continuous tear capsulotomy with every motion being made toward the incision.

The answer was yes: the pear-shaped capsulotomy (Figure 3-5). I think it is a wonderful and easy way to perform a continuous tear capsulotomy.

This technique begins with a Kellan disposable cystitome, which is available from Visitec. It is placed in the anterior capsule at the 6 o'clock position and pulled toward the incision. The shape of the cystitome is such that not only does it create a triangular flap immediately, but the apex of the triangle is rounded rather than pointed. As you pull the flap toward the incision, the flap becomes wider and wider (Figure 3-6). When it reaches the imaginary line between 10 o'clock and 2 o'clock, you stop pulling.

Use capsulotomy forceps to grab the anterior capsule near the tear at the 2 o'clock position and pull it toward 12 o'clock (Figure 3-7). Let go and grab the capsule at the 10 o'clock position and pull toward 12 o'clock (Figure 3-8). When the two tears meet, the capsulotomy is completed.

Three motions are made in this capsulotomy. Pulling the cystitome towards you, pulling one-half of the flap toward you, and then pulling the other half toward you. Three quick movements, all of

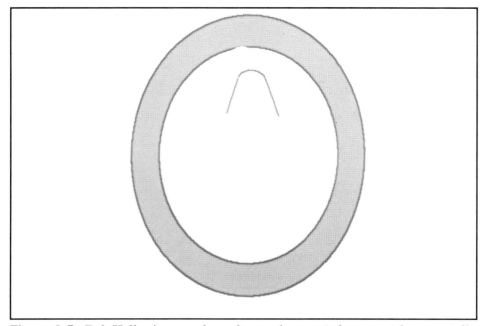

Figure 3-5. Bob Kellan's pear shaped capsulotomy is begun with a specially designed blunt cystitome that tears a triangular flap with a rounded apex.

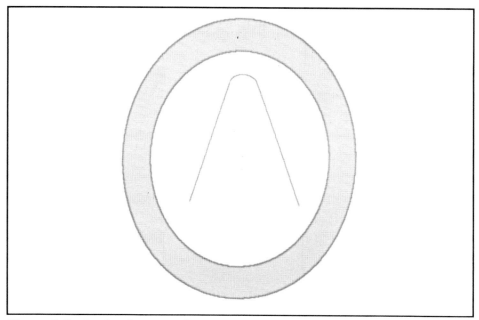

Figure 3-6. As the flap is pulled toward the incision with the cystitome, the flap becomes wider. When it reaches the line between 10 and 2 o'clock, the cystitome is exchanged for capsulotomy forceps.

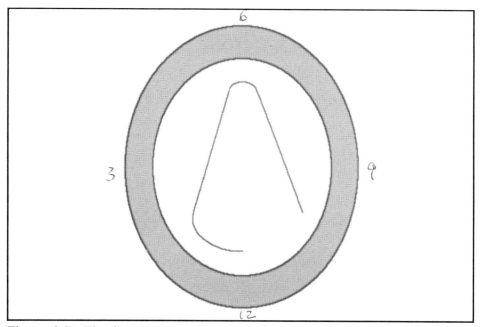

Figure 3-7. The flap is grasped with the forceps near the 2 o'clock position and torn to 12 o'clock.

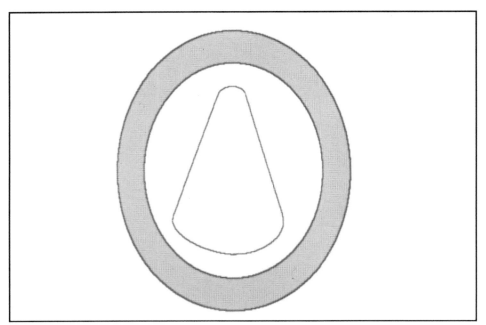

Figure 3-8. The flap is then grasped at 10 o'clock and torn back in to complete the capsulotomy at 12 o'clock.

them pulling something toward you, and you end up with a beautiful continuous tear capsulotomy. It is shaped something like a pear. Some people think it is shaped something like a Schmoo, a lovable creature from the old Li'l Abner cartoons.

Performing this capsulotomy is easy, but equally beneficial are some of the advantages of its shape. First of all, it is wider near the incision. That makes it easier to lift the superior pole of the nucleus (if necessary) and also easier to get out the superior cortex.

The inferior portion of the capsulotomy is narrow. This helps hold the nucleus down in the capsular bag when you are manipulating it and also gives clear anatomic landmarks for placing the inferior haptic of the intraocular lens even in eyes with miotic pupils.

All in all, I think this is a wonderful capsulotomy. If you are having difficulty making a circular capsulorhexis, I strongly urge you to try the pear-shaped capsulotomy.

Making the Transition

Taming the stray tear

Let's look at a few things that can happen during continuous tear capsulotomy that make its construction difficult. Suppose, for example, that you introduce a blunt cystitome into the eye, engage the anterior capsule and pull it toward the incision, but rather than getting a nice triangular flap you get a vertical slit (Figure 3-9). This is a bit of a problem. If you grab a vertical slit and try to make it tear, the slit will keep going straight to the equator (Figure 3-10). You need a curved tear in the anterior capsule before you can create a purposeful capsulotomy. If you find that the movement of your cystitome is causing a straight-line cut in the anterior capsule, then push your cystitome off to one side as you are pulling it toward the incision (Figure 3-11). Your straight-line cut then gets directed off to the side and becomes a gently curved one. The anterior capsule flap can be grasped with the forceps and the capsulotomy made easily as described above.

Suppose you begin the capsulotomy okay, but when you get to the 8 o'clock position the capsulotomy veers off toward the equator (Figure 3-12). How will you get that back on track again?

If the tear goes off just a little bit you can stop, regrasp and try to direct it down toward 6 o'clock. But if the direction of the tear is headed right for the equator, stop and do not go any further. Introduce fine scissors into the eye and make a snip at 8 o'clock, heading toward the 6 o'clock position of the anterior capsule. This will begin a new tear, and you can continue the capsulotomy anew (Figure 3-13).

What happens if you bring the capsulotomy around and when it gets to the 4 o'clock position it goes off course?

This time you have to start another capsulotomy at the 12 o'clock position (Figure 3-14). Make a snip in the anterior capsule toward the left, grab the new flap with forceps and tear it clockwise toward 4 o'clock, terminating this flap where the first one went off toward the equator (Figure 3-15).

As long as we are on the subject, why do tears go off to the equator anyway?

Picture a thin piece of material such as plastic food wrap. Imagine making a small round hole in that material and then from underneath taking something shaped like a cone, like a tent spike for example, and pushing it through the hole. When the point goes through the hole nothing happens because the point is smaller in

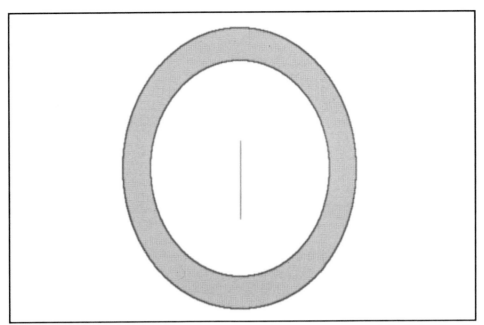

Figure 3-9. The creation of a vertical slit is one potential difficulty in beginning the capsulotomy with a blunt cystitome.

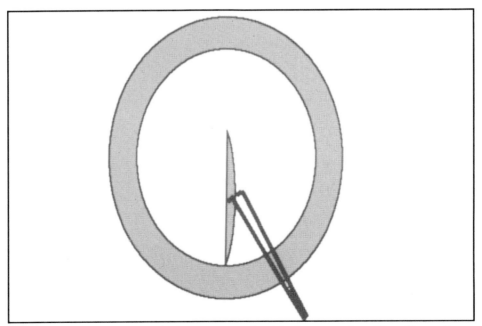

Figure 3-10. If a vertical slit is grasped with forceps, the slit will continue straight out to the equator.

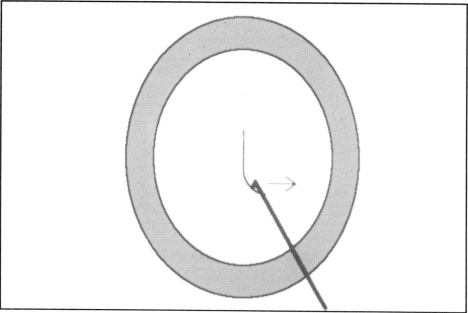

Figure 3-11. To correct a vertical slit, push the cystitome off to the side while pulling down toward the incision. The straight-line cut will become a gently curved one and you will be able to continue with forceps as previously described.

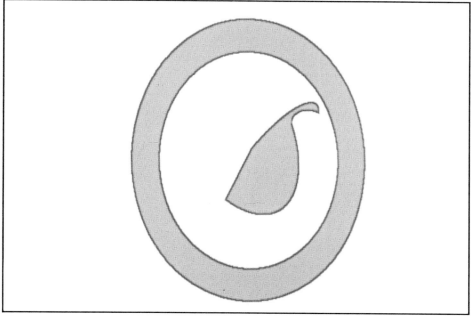

Figure 3-12. Occasionally the continuous tear capsulotomy will veer off toward the equator as it reaches the 8 o'clock position. If this happens, stop tearing with the forceps.

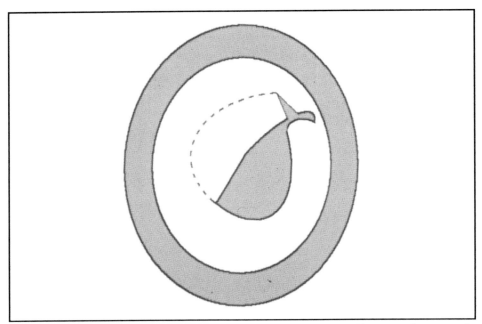

Figure 3-13. The tear can be redirected by making a small cut in the capsule with fine scissors. The capsulotomy is then continued with forceps.

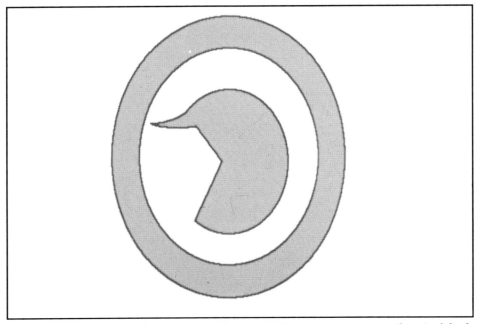

Figure 3-14. A tear that veers off toward the equator near the 4 o'clock position must also be halted immediately.

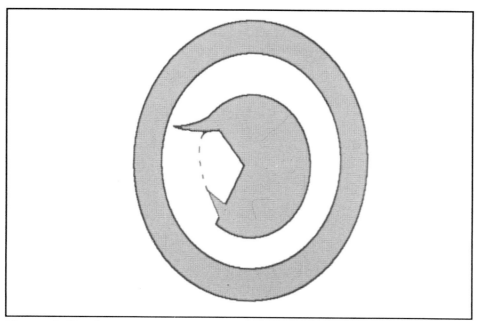

Figure 3-15. Scissors are again used, in this case to make a snip in the capsule toward 4 o'clock. The capsulotomy is then completed with forceps in a clockwise direction.

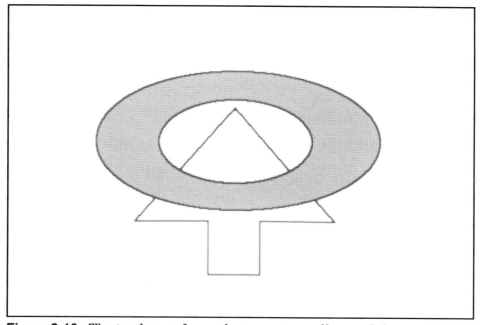

Figure 3-16. The tendency of capsular tears to go off toward the equator can be understood by imagining a conical object (here, an arrowhead) being forced up through a capsulotomy. Initially, the point of the cone will pass through the opening.

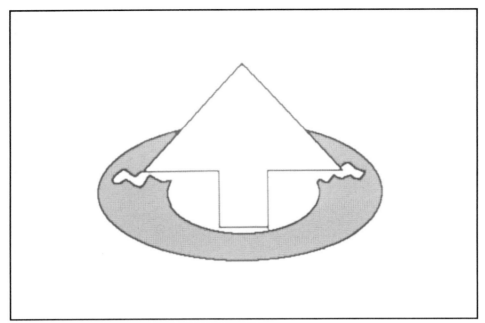

Figure 3-17. When a part of the cone with a diameter wider than the opening passes through the capsulotomy, the obvious result will be a tearing of the capsule toward the equator.

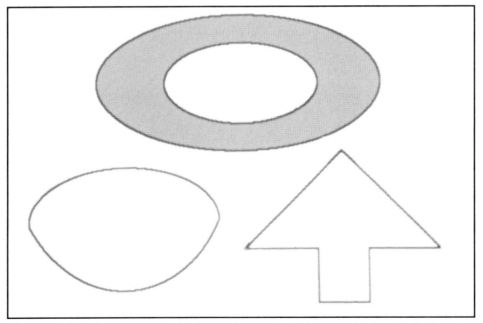

Figure 3-18. In a sense, the lens (lower left) is a conical object like the arrowhead (lower right). As the capsulotomy (top) is created, the lens pushes up through it, creating the tendency for the capsule to tear toward the equator.

diameter than the hole (Figure 3-16). But when a wider portion of the cone passes through where the diameter is bigger than the hole, the food wrap will split and tears will go off toward the periphery (Figure 3-17).

Now take that cone, round off the tip and repeat the experiment. The exact same thing happens. I know most of you see where I am going. A convex surface pressed against the food wrap will also eventually cause the central opening to split and tears to develop. The anterior surface of the lens nucleus is such a convex surface (Figure 3-18).

A lens pressing against the anterior capsule will encourage tears toward the equator. This imbalance in pressure is probably the most common cause for uncontrolled peripheral tearing. If you find you are getting such tears, or even if the diameter of the capsulotomy is simply larger than you want it to be, stop for a moment. Fill the anterior chamber with a viscoelastic and push down on the nucleus to take some of the pressure off the anterior capsule. You will be able to complete the capsulotomy easier, with fewer tears toward the periphery and with much more control.

In the process of grasping and regrasping the capsular flap during capsulorhexis, the handle of the forceps might lift the upper flap of the scleral incision and allow viscoelastic to escape. If you see this happening early on, you should again stop, inject more viscoelastic and then resume the capsulotomy.

Discussion

Importance of capsulorhexis

There are two reasons why the continuous tear capsulotomy is important. Forget what you might have heard about intraocular lens centration and ensuring placement of the haptics inside the bag. These things are true, but they are not the most important things.

The single most important reason why the continuous tear capsulotomy is important is that it holds the nucleus down in the capsular bag during phacoemulsification. It changes the entire operation by limiting where the nucleus can go and, more importantly, by limiting where your phaco tip must go. It forces you to keep the tip in the bag and working on the nucleus. It does not let you wander around the anterior chamber wreaking all sorts of havoc.

The second reason why the continuous tear capsulotomy is so important is because it helps to maintain a nearly intact capsular bag. This capsulotomy only opens a window into the anterior capsule. The structural rigidity and integrity of the capsular bag are nearly identical to a completely intact bag. This is a very important concept. It makes every principle in this book the opposite of what we discussed in previous editions. The operation is entirely different from the one we did with a can opener capsulotomy.

With a can opener capsulotomy the anterior capsule was peeled back, leaving an irregular ridge of tissue. The purpose of the can opener capsulotomy was to permit the nucleus to get out of the bag. It was designed to destroy the integrity of the bag. The continuous tear capsulotomy is just the opposite. It preserves the integrity of the bag to hold the nucleus inside.

That is why converting to nucleus expression during phacoemulsification is so much more difficult now than it used to be. Prolapsing the nucleus through a continuous tear capsulotomy would be fraught with difficulties. For all practical purposes, we must consider the can opener capsulotomy to be associated with nucleus expression and iris plane phacoemulsification. The continuous tear capsulotomy to be associated with in-the-bag phacoemulsification. Of course there are exceptions—but we cannot permit too much leeway.

Converting to extracapsular procedure

Capsulorhexis is a commitment to endocapsular phaco. And as Bob Kellan says in our course, if you break the commitment you have to break the capsulorhexis.

If you are converting to extracap after doing some sculpting of the nucleus, two relaxing scissor cuts should be made in the capsule at the 10:30 and 1:30 positions. The cuts will provide an opening in the capsule wide enough for the lens to pass through.

Visibility of the capsulorhexis edge may be a problem. When the red reflex is lost, a viscoelastic can make the capsule easier to see. Usually, however, you will know where the capsulorhexis is and be able to snip it with the scissors.

Preserving bag structure

Even an extremely delicate cataract surgical technique produces stretching of zonular fibers and traction on the ciliary body. When you see the lens move during phaco, you are looking at some degree of capsular shift and zonular stretch. The closer the phaco tip comes to the capsule, the greater is the potential for a capsule tear.

Zonular dehiscence can lead to implant malposition or dislocation intraoperatively or late in postoperative course; possible protrusion of a lens haptic through the bag; and potential for large posterior capsule tears in the long term, especially during the capsular bag contraction that occurs with normal healing.

Gentle, controlled movements during phaco, careful attention during aspiration and patience during the irrigation and aspiration of cortical material are the keys to maintaining the capsule and zonules. A surprising amount of tension and stress is exerted on the zonules during I&A, particularly as the probe approaches the equator of the capsule to remove cortex from its attachments to the bag. Normal zonules usually rebound readily, however.

Both the capsule and the zonules are elastic. David Apple's group at the Center for Intraocular Lens Research measured the overall natural elasticity at about 1.5 mm for the capsule and zonules. On average, the structure will withstand a net 3 mm stretch and rebound without breaking. This action will come into play when we look at the phacoemulsification of the nucleus, especially when we discuss the relaxing nucleotomy maneuver.

Physiologic trampoline

After many years of performing phacoemulsification using techniques that stretched and distorted the capsular bag—techniques such as anterior chamber phaco, iris plane phaco, and for that matter anything that uses a can opener capsulotomy—we are all learning and appreciating the value of the continuous tear capsulotomy. One of the truly impressive features of a continuous tear capsulotomy is that the capsule is left essentially intact and tends to have very good structural rigidity.

With the can opener capsulotomy, you can move the nucleus in the capsular bag to a very large degree. This was necessary in trying to prolapse the nucleus for anterior chamber phacoemulsification, for example. Those of us accustomed to performing phacoemulsification using a can opener capsulotomy need to learn the limits of capsular bag tolerance as they are established with the continuous tear capsulotomy. One thing is clear. If you have a continuous tear capsulotomy, the anterior capsule will not give way to accommodate very much movement of the nucleus. Excessive movement will tear the capsule or the zonules.

I like to look at the nearly intact capsular bag and the zonular ring as a physiologic trampoline. The capsular bag is the fabric and the zonules are the springs of the trampoline. They can accommodate small displacements of the nucleus by shifting and stretching, and when one releases the nucleus, everything springs back to the usual position.

It is important to realize that the amount the nucleus can move within the bag depends on the density of the nucleus. If the cataract is very dense, it may be moved only a very small amount, perhaps a millimeter or so. If the cataract is soft and there is a lot of give within the nuclear lamellae, it may be able to move a few millimeters.

When performing phacoemulsification in the capsular bag, one must respect the physiologic trampoline at all times and not perform any maneuvers which unnecessarily distort or interfere with its functions.

For example, if you want to emulsify a portion of the nucleus at 6 o'clock, you could leave the nucleus in place and push the phaco tip to the periphery of the nucleus. Usually this is not a good idea. The tip could disappear under the inferior iris. You might even pass the phaco tip through the capsular bag itself. A better strategy would be to begin to emulsify the inferior nucleus, then hold the phaco tip still and permit the inferior nucleus to "follow" to the tip. (Even in 1991 we have not forgotten the concept of followability.)

If the nucleus moves superiorly as the inferior nucleus follows into the tip, you can imagine the stresses placed on the physiologic trampoline. As the nucleus moves superiorly, it presses tightly against the superior capsule, stretching the capsular bag first and then the inferior zonules. If the nucleus continues to be aspirated vigorously toward the tip, something will have to give. Either the nucleus will pop through the superior capsule or the inferior zonules will break.

If, on the other hand, more moderate amounts of aspiration are used with the emulsification, or if the emulsification is performed in the pulse mode, the nucleus will come superiorly only until the superior capsule and the inferior zonules are stretched to a physiologic limit. The nucleus will then spring away from the phaco tip by the action of the physiologic trampoline. The nucleus will separate itself from the phaco tip and return to its usual position, leaving the capsular bag and zonular ring intact.

By recognizing the actions of the physiologic trampoline we can work in the capsular bag with virtual impunity. It becomes very unlikely that we will accidentally break the posterior capsule or the zonules, thus enhancing the ease and efficacy of the operation and improving benefits to the patient.

4

Hydrodissection

I can remember a time when we made a whole list of reasons why hydrodissection is important. I have thrown away that list. I now believe there is only one reason to perform hydrodissection: to make it possible to rotate the nucleus.

Hydrodissection breaks the cortical adhesions so that the nucleus becomes free-floating in the capsular bag. It can be rotated to bring different parts of the nucleus to the 6 o'clock position so they can be worked on and emulsified in the capsular bag.

We never liked doing hydrodissection when we used iris plane phacoemulsification. In the second edition of this book, the cortical attachments were even called "the third hand" in phaco. In the context of a can-opener capsulotomy technique, that third hand was absolutely necessary. We needed something to hold onto the nucleus while we sculpted it. We needed the cortical adhesions because the can opener capsulotomy permitted the nucleus to come up into the anterior chamber. That also meant that later on we had to do superior pole prolapse and a bunch of other maneuvers to break the cortical adhesions.

Now that we are doing in-the-bag phacoemulsification and continuous tear capsulotomy, the nucleus cannot come forward into the anterior chamber. We are free to loosen it as much as we want in

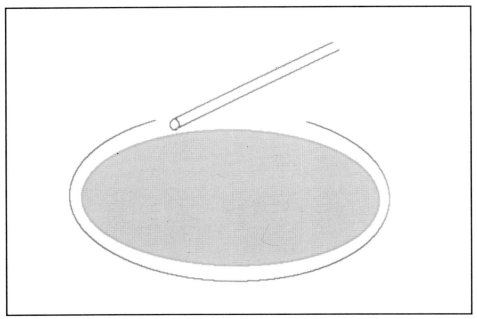

Figure 4-1. In hydrodissection, balanced salt solution is injected under the anterior capsule flap.

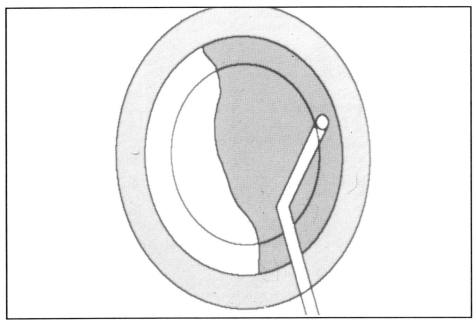

Figure 4-2. It is important that the fluid dissects around the equator, flows underneath the nucleus, and separates the nucleus from its cortical attachments. If the fluid wave is not seen and the nucleus does not move, then hydrodissection has not been performed.

order to make the operation as easy as possible. And that is why hydrodissection is important. Please do not let anyone talk you into believing that it is any more difficult or sophisticated than that.

Hydrodissection is the injection of balanced salt solution under the anterior capsule flap (Figure 4-1) until the fluid dissects around the equator, flows underneath the nucleus, and separates the nucleus from its cortical attachments (Figure 4-2). If you do not see the fluid wave and if the nucleus does not move, then you do not have hydrodissection. You might have done a fluid rinse but you have not done a dissection of the nucleus from its cortical attachments.

Please keep in mind the word dissection. It is critical here.

Injecting fluid without achieving dissection of the nucleus is not hydrodissection. There must be definite plane separation between the nucleus and the cortical debris that remains attached to the capsular bag. If you do not see the fluid wave and if the nucleus does not move, then simply replace the cannula in another position and do it again. One place where adhesions like to remain is at 12 o'clock, so you might need to go in through the side port and squirt up under the anterior capsule at the 12 o'clock position. Keep in mind that until the nucleus can rotate freely in the capsular bag, the dissection has not been completed.

Technique

Hydrodissection

I used to use a 30-gauge cannula for hydrodissection, but found much better results with larger sizes of 25 to 27 gauge. The tip of the cannula I use is sharpened, somewhat like an Atkinson needle, to facilitate the second hydro step that follows hydrodissection.

The cannula is placed on a 3-cc syringe filled with BSS. The tip of the cannula is passed under the anterior capsulotomy after completion of the capsulorhexis. A minimal amount of fluid is injected, and a "muffling" of the red reflex will usually occur. You do not want to inject too much fluid. You can do thorough hydrodissection and second hydro (our next step, which we'll get to in a minute) and only inject about 1 or 2 cc of BSS.

The next step has been called hydrodelamination, hydrodelineation and hydrodemarcation. It is all the same stuff and I just refer to it as the other hydro step: the injection of balanced salt solution into the body of the nucleus to try to separate out an inner nucleus from an outer nucleus. This whole idea of inner and outer nucleus is a new concept in cataract anatomy and one that we should spend some time on. We had a whole chapter on the structural considerations of incisions, and I think we also need to spend quite a bit of time on the concentric anatomy of the lens. Let's go on to that next.

The concentric anatomy of the lens

For purposes of this discussion I want you to forget what you've learned about the fetal nucleus and the adult nucleus. What I want to talk about is similar but not exactly the same, so I want to start off with a blank slate.

The lens in cross section is made up of a concentric series of elliptical rings. Each one of these rings represents growth of the lens and the laying down of additional lens material from the epithelial cells located on the underside of the anterior capsule. Where else have we seen concentric rings laid down by growth? The most common place we see such a pattern is in trees. If we cut down a tree we see a series of rings, each representing one year of growth. There are a couple of principles I want to bring out using a tree as an analogy for a cataract.

Pines and oaks

In my back yard we have a lot of pine trees. I watch these trees when a storm is raging outside, and they sway back and forth in the breeze. They bend and flex as the wind hits them. If I go out and grab a pine tree branch and try to break it, it bends until it forms a hairpin loop. If I cut a pine tree, the inside of it will be moist with oozings of sap. The concentric lamellae of tree tissue are widely spaced, and if I touch the inside of the branch the tissue is moist.

I want you to accept the pine tree as an analogy for a soft or medium density cataract. The concentric lamellae of cataract tissue are not densely packed, so much of the space inside the cataract is taken up by moisture. (I do not know if this is 100% anatomically accurate or not, but it helps me to think this way. I hope it will help you to think of cataracts this way as well.) For purposes of this discussion I am going to define the soft and medium cataract as having the same characteristics of a pine tree, so I will call these cataracts pine tree cataracts.

In my front yard we have a lot of oak trees, and when a storm blows they make an awful mess. Twigs and branches fall down and mess up my lawn. If I look out the window and watch the tree during a storm the tree sways back and forth, but as soon as it moves as much as it can, branches will crack and fall to the ground. If later on I go out and examine these branches, I can see that the concentric lamellae of tree tissue are densely packed and feel dry. If I take an oak tree branch and bend it, it will snap and break. It is impossible to take an oak tree branch and bend it into a hairpin. Oak trees have a natural tendency to crack and break rather than to bend and flex.

I am going to suggest that medium to firm density cataracts have characteristics of an oak tree, so I am going to call them oak tree cataracts. These cataracts have concentric lamellae of tissue that are densely packed together, packed so tight that there is no room for moisture between lamellae. There is no capacity for normal elasticity, so if you try to bend or flex these cataracts they will snap.

The pine tree and the oak tree have very dissimilar reactions to the forces presented during a storm. Pine tree cataracts and oak tree cataracts likewise have very different reactions to the forces presented during phacoemulsification. They respond differently, so the forces need to be applied differently. It only makes sense to individualize the operation to take advantage of the natural tendencies of each type of cataract.

If we are operating on a pine tree cataract, we are going to want to have an operation that emphasizes bending and flexing. If we are operating on an oak tree cataract, we want to have an operation that emphasizes breaking and cracking.

In the next few chapters we will be discussing different surgical strategies for handling these two types of cataracts. We will use spring surgery as a model of the operations that emphasize bending and flexing for pine tree cataracts, and we will use four-quadrant cracking as a model for operations that emphasize breaking and cracking for the oak tree cataracts. But before we jump into phaco techniques, let's get back to our hydro steps.

In theory anyway, it ought to be possible to separate the cataract into a series of wafer thin rings by injecting fluid between each layer, allowing it to float freely from the others. This is the goal of such fluid dissection techniques as nuclear hydrolysis and hydrosonics. For the techniques we will be discussing, however, only two fluid planes are necessary. We already created the first fluid plane by hydrodissection. The second plane will be created with the other hydro step.

There is one good reason to do second hydro: to isolate the hard inner part of the cataract. That's the part that needs to be phacoemulsified. The rest of it will come out with aspiration, saving you time and sparing the eye from unnecessary ultrasound.

The other hydro step

You start the other hydro step by pushing the cannula right into the body of the nucleus until it meets resistance. That resistance is a rather poorly defined point where soft peripheral cataract tissue meets hard central cataract tissue. We can define it as a place where the outer nucleus meets the inner nucleus. The tip will pass through the soft outer nucleus and stop when it hits the hard part of the cataract (Figure 4-3). I have never seen a case where it was possible to push the cannula right through the whole lens to the posterior capsule.

Upon injecting fluid, the "golden ring" will signal the true separation of nuclear layers (Figure 4-4). With a small cataract you will see a ring about 7 mm in diameter. I do not think there is any advantage to hydrolyzing the nucleus extensively. You end up giving yourself more work by creating all of these individual layers of nucleus to emulsify one at a time. It is enough to just separate the inner and outer layers.

There is one exception to performing both hydrodissection and the other hydro step. In younger patients (anyone under the age of 50), it is easier if you perform only hydrodissection. The nucleus will be soft and will follow into the phaco tip easily. If you only do hydrodissection, the entire body of the nucleus will be emulsified easily. If you have performed the other hydro step, you can easily remove a small inner nucleus but run the risk of being stuck with a thick outer nuclear shell adherent to the capsular bag. You will find it difficult to manipulate that shell because it is so soft your spatula will move right through it. You will not be able to get a purchase on it and will

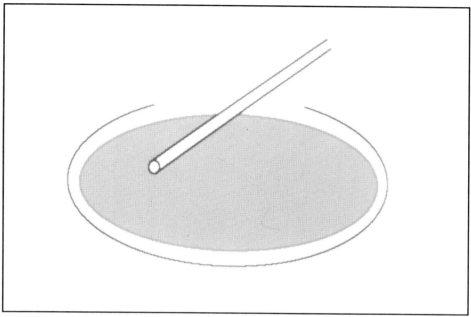

Figure 4-3. The second hydro step begins with the cannula being pushed into the body of the nucleus until it meets resistance. This will be at the point where soft peripheral cataract tissue meets hard central cataract tissue: where the outer nucleus meets the inner nucleus.

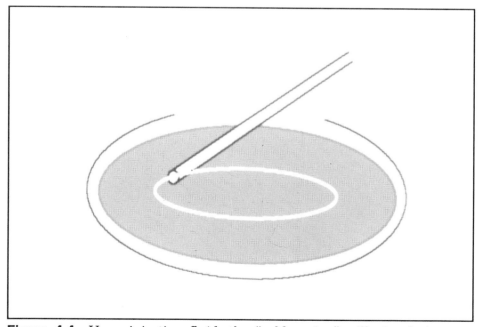

Figure 4-4. Upon injecting fluid, the "golden ring" will signal the true separation of nuclear layers. With a small cataract, the ring will be about 7 mm in diameter.

end up doing extensive aspiration with the wide phaco tip. That is very dangerous and just too much work. Please take my advice and do only hydrodissection in very soft cataracts and especially if a patient is under 50 years old.

Discussion

There is nothing magic about an inner or an outer nucleus. It is a relative term describing the densities of the nucleus. The sizes of the "inner" and "outer" nucleus depend on the nature of the cataract. Harder cataracts will have a larger core. This inner nucleus (some people call it an endonucleus) is hard and firm. The outer nucleus is soft. Some people call it the cortical zone or the peripheral nuclear lamellae. The phraseology is not important. What is important is the concept that within the cataract there is a point where you can make a fluid dissection, isolating an inner nucleus from an outer nucleus.

This is a very important concept, because the dangerous part of the nucleus is the inner nucleus. The inner nucleus is firm and hard. If you cut it, you can get a sharp edge that can damage the posterior capsule. The inner nucleus is hard in the sense of firmness, and it is hard in the sense of being the most difficult part of the cataract to remove. By contrast the outer nucleus is a pussycat. It can be removed almost with aspiration, although most of the time a little bit of emulsification power is necessary to get it out easily.

By separating the inner and outer nucleus, the outer nucleus can serve as a shell within which we will emulsify the inner nucleus. You can think of the outer nucleus as something like a foam rubber cushion that sits between the posterior capsule and the inner nucleus, effectively isolating it. If a sharp edge of inner nucleus goes out of control, it will cut the outer nucleus rather than the posterior capsule. If your phaco tip moves suddenly for whatever reason, it will fall away from the inner nucleus into the outer cushion rather than falling through the posterior capsule into the vitreous.

I think that hydrodissection and the other hydro step should be performed in every cataract operation (with the exception of young, soft cataracts, as stated). These steps should be performed because they help to isolate the inner nucleus for safety of removal and because they break all the adhesions within the capsular bag, permitting tissue to come to the tip easily.

If you bring your phaco tip near the capsular bag, there is a potential for the capsule to be aspirated. If you have performed a good fluid dissection, however, there is almost no tendency for the capsule to follow into the tip when you remove pieces of the nucleus because they are not attached. They have been dissected from each other.

5

Phacoemulsification Terminology: Six Basic Maneuvers

The development of the continuous tear capsulotomy changed the way we look at cataract surgery.

Back when we used a can-opener capsulotomy we had a lot of options when it came to removing the nucleus. The capsulotomy opened easily and permitted the nucleus to come out of the capsular bag. The capsulotomy was suitable both for nucleus expression and for iris plane phacoemulsification. The continuous tear capsulotomy changed all that. One of the specific features of this capsulotomy is that it holds the nucleus down in a nearly intact capsular bag. Our options for removing the nucleus become limited, for all practical purposes, to phacoemulsification in the bag.

Several different endocapsular techniques have evolved, differing primarily in whether they advocate cracking of the posterior plates. Howard Gimbel began this movement with his Divide and Conquer technique. But, just as all cataracts are not the same, all endocapsular procedures need not be the same either. Not all cataracts need to be divided, nor do they need to be conquered. Trying to decide the appropriate technique for a particular cataract puts us in the dilemma of the endocapsular egg. To crack, or not to crack?

Oak trees and pines

Remember how we compared cataracts to trees in Chapter 4? Both trees and cataracts are made up of concentric lamellae. The cataract's lamellae are pressed together tightly by the progressive laying down of new tissue within the confines of the capsular bag.

We divided cataracts into two types: pine-tree cataracts (loosely packed lamellae, moist, flexible, soft) and oak-tree cataracts (tightly packed lamellae, drier, brittle, hard). These two extremes can serve as a model for the two types of endocapsular phacoemulsification, the cracking and the non-cracking techniques.

The analysis of the nucleus begins during sculpting. The amount of tissue removed with each pass varies with the density of the nucleus and the relationship between the nuclear lamellae and nuclear hydration.

Evaluating the nucleus

As a general guideline, if more than half a needle's width of tissue can be removed with a single pass of the phaco tip, the nucleus is reasonably loose and hydrated. This is the sign of a pine tree cataract. If less than a quarter of a needle's width of tissue can be removed with each pass, the nucleus is denser, with a lower water content. This is a sign of an oak tree cataract.

If you have a pine tree cataract, you must consider the spring surgery strategy of flexing the nucleus so the nuclear segments bend in towards the middle of the capsular bag. This can be done only if there is room for them, so deep and broad sculpting has to be carried out. For this technique to be performed on an oak tree cataract, the posterior plate has to be very, very thin because the posterior plate of an oak tree cataract has very little give to it—it would rather break than bend.

This being the case, it makes little sense to try to flex the sides in. Instead the nuclear segments should be nudged apart, and the dense, dry lamellae will separate easily, breaking the nucleus into smaller pieces.

The dilemma of the endocapsular egg, to crack or not to crack, can be solved by appreciating the differences in the stretch and bend characteristics of the nucleus. The densely packed, dry nucleus—what I've referred to as an oak tree nucleus—cracks easily. Working with, rather than against nature, suggests that we perform a cracking procedure. The looser, more hydrated cataract—what I've referred to as a pine tree cataract—resists cracking but cooperates with bending and flexing. Therefore, a non-cracking technique would be preferred.

Selecting the appropriate phacoemulsification approach to each individual cataract makes the operation safer, more likely to be successful, and less likely to be associated with intraoperative complications. For some cataracts we must answer ... To crack? Yes. For others, not to crack? Yes.

The six essential phaco maneuvers

In order to properly discuss various endocapsular phacoemulsification techniques, we need a common language, terms and phrases which describe various steps common the endocapsular techniques now being used. Terms like the carousel, the ice cream scoop, and lollipop do not have much relevance today. Maneuvers taking place within the capsular bag are different and require different terminology.

New terminology is also necessary for students of endocapsular phacoemulsification so that they can learn the essential phacoemulsification maneuvers and be able to practice them in the laboratory.

After reviewing all of the major techniques of endocapsular phacoemulsification, I find that there are six maneuvers which are common to all or most of them: sculpting, trench digging, relaxing nucleotomy, peripheral aspiration and removal (PAAR), posterior plate shaving and nuclear cracking.

Sculpting. The first and oldest posterior chamber phacoemulsification maneuver maintains its role of prominence in the endocapsular techniques. Regardless of the method used, sculpting remains the easiest and safest step of the operation. Sculpting also remains the single most potent force in phacoemulsification.

For this reason, I am somewhat puzzled by those who minimize its role in some techniques. Some surgeons prefer to carve out a little notch in the nucleus and then try to split it. Is the charm of a nucleus crack distractive from the gentle joy of sculpting a nucleus?

The sculpting varies from technique to technique, ranging from the large craters of spring surgery and chip-and-flip to the more narrow trenches of four quarter cracking and fractional phaco. However, regardless of the shape, or the size, or the depth of sculpting, it remains the most important step of all phacoemulsification techniques.

Sculpting is a high-power maneuver. A common mistake in beginning phaco is to shy away from high power levels. That is one of the worst things to do. You end up bludgeoning the cataract instead of cutting it. If you see a nucleus rocking back and forth, you are not using enough power.

I advocate aggressive central sculpting because it is the easiest maneuver to perform and it removes the hardest part of the nucleus.

Trench digging. Some techniques involve the production of trenches as the primary method of dividing the nucleus. Others use trenching as an adjunct to other methods, as to assist in the preparation of a relaxing nucleotomy (see below).

Trench digging produces a groove in the nucleus into which can be passed the phaco tip or other instruments, including crackers and dividers. A trench is typically about two tip diameters wide at the top, narrower at the bottom, and extends out to the cleavage plane between the inner and the outer nucleus.

Trenches are usually made in firm central nuclear tissue, and so are developed with reasonably high phaco power during the rough outline stages, and then with lower levels of phaco power when working near the periphery or posterior portions of the nucleus.

The "feel" during trench digging is very much like sculpting, except that a less expansive technique is called for. In sculpting the goal is to clean out the whole nucleus, so material is removed liberally. In trench digging, every stoke must be kept within the zone two phaco tips wide and three deep. This is wide enough to get two instruments in and crack the nucleus, and it leaves enough peripheral nucleus for the instruments to push against without slicing through.

Relaxing nucleotomy. Similar to a relaxing incision, a relaxing nucleotomy produces a slit which permits tissues to move easily.

A relaxing nucleotomy is usually made in the inner nuclear girdle to facilitate removal of the girdle itself. Until the nucleotomy is performed, the inner nuclear girdle is a firm ring which is unable to collapse in on itself. The ring sits under the anterior capsule peripheral to the capsulorhexis opening.

If the inner nuclear girdle can be split, the structural integrity of the round structure will be lost and all of its elements will be free to move.

A relaxing nucleotomy is no more than a small trench which creates a through and through opening between the area of sculpting and the cleavage plane between the inner and the outer nucleus, permitting the tissue on either side of it to collapse in towards the middle of the capsular bag.

The relaxing nucleotomy is the maneuver where we break the rigid structure of the lens so we can fold it in spring surgery, the subject of the next chapter.

Posterior plate shaving. Whether the nucleus is to be cracked into pieces or collapsed in towards the middle of the bag, the procedure is facilitated when the posterior plate is thin. A thin plate requires only a nudge to crack it apart, minimizing the outward effort required. A thin plate also folds easier than a thick one, acting more like a willow branch rather than a dried twig.

Posterior plate shaving can be part of other phacoemulsification maneuvers. It can be part of sculpting, making the sculpted area as deep as possible. It can be part of trench digging or of a relaxing nucleotomy.

However it is used, posterior plate shaving needs to be performed gently, using low phaco power, for maximum control. If the passes are limited to approximately the thickness of the wall of the phaco needle it is possible, for example, to shave the nucleus into two pieces by shaving right down and into the cleavage plane present before the thin layer of outer nucleus is reached.

This is the maneuver that inspires fear. People are afraid that they cannot tell how deep the tip is going, and afraid that the next stroke will tear through the posterior capsule.

When emulsifying the posterior layers of nucleus near the capsule, you obviously do not want to take full-bore bites of tissue like you do in central sculpting. Instead, shave very thin layers barely as thick as the wall of the phaco tip. You will not push the tip through the posterior capsule if you shave along the lamellae of the cataract in this way.

It is not a blind maneuver, since the tip should not be going under the iris. You can see the grayish nuclear material that has to be removed. So long as there is lens tissue visible, the capsule is safe. When you shave down an area one tip wide to where the red reflex shows through, that serves as a guide for the thickness of the rest of the posterior plate.

Sometimes it is necessary to lift the posterior plate away from the capsule. This can be accomplished in a combination maneuver by simultaneously shaving and drawing the phaco tip up away from the capsule. Once the plate is thin enough, it will flex much more easily. This is much more easily accomplished with a diaphragm or venturi type of aspiration rather than a peristaltic machine. Peristaltic pumps have to be pretty well occluded before suction builds up, although a sweeping motion toward the fornix with the bevel sideways can help you get enough of a grip on the nucleus to pull it away from the capsule.

Peripheral aspiration and removal (PAAR). The portions of the nucleus under the anterior capsule have to be gathered up and brought away from the capsule before they can be easily visualized and safely removed. This holds true whether the pieces are the nuclear rim of Chip & Flip, the nuclear quarters of Four Quadrant Phaco or Fractional Phaco, or the nuclear handles (the semi-hemi nuclei) of spring surgery.

Peripheral Aspiration and Removal is a descriptive term which indicates that a portion of nucleus is aspirated with the phaco tip, drawn inwards and away from the capsular fornix, and emulsified safely.

This is made easier by turning the phaco tip sideways, so the capsule is less likely to occlude the tip and be torn.

It takes discipline not to apply phaco power immediately upon grasping the peripheral nucleus. The nuclear material must be drawn into the center of the bag for emulsification, however. This is a safety mechanism that will be absolutely essential to performing phaco by nuclear cracking techniques. Speaking of which, the last of our six basic maneuvers is....

Nuclear cracking. I'm not forgetting about this "phaco" maneuver. In fact, you'll see a whole chapter on nuclear cracking.

Making the Transition

Practicing the six essential phaco maneuvers

The limitations of teaching nuclear rotation, superior pole iris prolapse, and so forth are well known. Instructors often had to admonish students not to worry because human eyes were much easier to work on than the laboratory eyes.

These limitations are not a problem with these basic phaco maneuvers. I feel that model eyes and animal eyes are better suited to practicing the maneuvers of in-the-bag phaco than iris-plane phaco. Each of the basic maneuvers can be learned on the soft cataracts of animal eyes or the hard plastic nuclei of model eyes. As a result, wet labs are more representative of real surgery and thereby can be more productive.

Describing a surgical technique

Now that we have a common terminology, we can describe a particular technique very clearly using the six basic steps. We'll be looking at spring surgery in the next chapter, which can be described as: wide and deep sculpting, inferior relaxing nucleotomy, three hours of PAAR, a single 180° rotation, completion of sculpting, another inferior relaxing nucleotomy, three more hours of PAAR, posterior plate shaving, then PAAR of the two remaining sections of inner nuclear girdle.

Of course, there's just a little bit more to say about spring surgery. For example, why is it called *spring*?

6

Spring Surgery

Spring surgery is a form of endocapsular phacoemulsification that I find very simple to understand and easy to perform. It is my usual method for removing soft and medium density cataracts, and it is the method which I suggest you learn if you want to convert from nucleus expression procedures to phacoemulsification.

I consider spring surgery a basic phaco technique that should be used for pine-tree cataracts. It evolved from Howard Fine's chip-and-flip method, in which the key element is the separation of inner and outer sections of nucleus. That's what we did with our two hydro steps. The unique part of spring surgery is the shaping of the nucleus into two handles that can be pulled down into the bag and emulsified.

The name spring has two meanings. One has to do with the natural springing action of the physiologic trampoline we talked about in chapter 3: the capsular bag and zonular ring. SPRING is also an acronym for Sequential Pulsed Removal of the Inner Nuclear Girdle. The nuclear girdle is a structure we create by the two hydro maneuvers followed by sculpting of the central nucleus.

Technique

The phaco tip is inserted bevel-down to pass easily over the iris and then is rotated 180°.

The superior-inferior motion of the globe is an indication of how tightly the probe fits into the incision. A good incision will be just wide enough to allow the probe to slide in and out without making the eye move up and down at all.

In a similar way, the motion of the nucleus tells you if you are using enough phaco power during sculpting. If the tip has enough power to cut through the cataract, the nucleus will not move around a lot while you sculpt it. If you do see the nucleus moving around in the eye, you are not using enough power. The tip is pushing the cataract instead of cutting it.

Five-zone approach

The strategy of spring surgery is to consider the nucleus to be made up of five zones: one central zone and four girdle zones. (This description is illustrated in the special section of color drawings that begins immediately after this chapter. All of the references to figure numbers are for that section.)

The central zone is removed using deep and relatively broad sculpting (Figure 2). Spring surgery is partly based on the premise that sculpting remains the easiest, most effective way to remove nuclear tissue. If you are not aggressive enough in sculpting the nucleus, you could end up with a very thick, firm bowl that is hard to manipulate. You must also avoid the opposite extreme, however, of sculpting yourself into a corner, where only a thin, unmanageable nuclear shell is left.

Good sculpting will leave you with a firm, structurally intact girdle of inner nucleus. This girdle will be outlined by the hydro cleavage plane between the inner and outer nucleus and defined on the inside by the extent of your sculpting. It is similar to the girdle of a hollow tree stump, and must be broken so we can collapse the nucleus into the bag for safe emulsification. The girdle is broken by making a pair of relaxing nucleotomies.

The phaco tip is placed on the inferior nucleus at the 6 o'clock position. The relaxing nucleotomy should be made (on average) around the inferior two clock hours of the nucleus about 2 mm deep (or twice the width of the phaco tip; see Figure 3). You have to keep the tip near the edge of the capsulotomy rather than going down into the capsular fornix. Let the nuclear material come to the tip during this maneuver rather than moving the tip further down into the bag. You should need only a low level of aspiration. Pulsed power makes the job easier, but if you do not have a pulse mode on your machine you can use a series of light taps on the foot pedal to apply bursts of minimal linear power.

There is little danger of aspirating capsule during this maneuver, even though the tip of the probe is very close to the capsulotomy edge. The posterior capsule will not follow the lens material into the port because we separated the tissues with hydrodissection.

The margin of safety during relaxing nucleotomy is not infinitely wide, however, and we have some pretty clear signals when we cross it. Recall the concept of the physiologic trampoline.

When you hold the phaco tip at the inferior part of the inner nucleus and aspirate it, the contents of the capsular bag move up, exerting a stretch on the inferior zonules. Pressure is also directed superiorly when the rigid inner nucleus moves toward the tip, compressing the cleavage plane between the hydrodissected nuclear layers. The inferior zonules pull back on the nucleus. When the tension in the zonules overcomes the force of aspiration, there is a natural rebound of the nucleus away from the tip. The result is that the nucleus will normally "chug" back and forth toward the stationary phaco tip.

Be alert for a deviation from this pattern during the relaxing nucleotomy. If the nucleus keeps coming toward the phaco tip and does not move back to the center of the bag, even when you switch off the aspiration, the zonules have been broken. Once you remove enough of the nucleus, however, the compressive forces are not present and the trampoline will not have the same pressure on it. The lens will cease to rebound away from the tip. The important thing to remember is that zonular rupture is not likely to occur during relaxing nucleotomy with pulse mode and low aspiration settings, so long as the phaco tip is held steady.

The next step is peripheral aspiration and removal (PAAR) of the two to three clock hours of the inner nuclear girdle adjacent to the relaxing nucleotomy (Figure 4). The PAAR maneuver, as you recall from the last chapter, involves aspirating the nucleus with the phaco tip, drawing it centrally (away from the capsule) and emulsifying it safely in the middle of the bag. We use this maneuver to widen the area of the relaxing nucleotomy, creating two distinct handles of nucleus with enough room between them for the handles to be folded inward.

After PAAR of several clock hours of inner nuclear girdle, the nucleus is rotated 180° (Figure 5). For all practical purposes, this single 180° rotation is the only rotation maneuver performed during this operation. It is just about the only time the second instrument is needed. After rotation, another relaxing nucleotomy is made (Figure 6) and several clock hours of inner nucleus are removed (Figure 7) using the same maneuvers.

What's left now are our two nuclear handles separated by a thin plate of posterior nucleus. This central portion of the nuclear plate is shaved some more until it is very thin (Figure 8). Now the two nuclear handles can be aspirated, pulled into the middle of the capsular bag, and emulsified (Figures 9 and 10).

The PAAR maneuver is again utilized. Unlike the nuclear cracking techniques, which push outward on the capsular bag when the nuclear segments are separated, the PAAR maneuver of spring surgery pulls the nuclear segments in toward the middle of the bag.

The creation of the nuclear handles is what prevents the formation of a thin outer nuclear shell. We did not sculpt the nucleus around its entire circumference. We removed tissue at opposite ends of the inner nucleus, maintaining the sides of the nucleus to leave some tissue for manipulation.

When the inner nucleus is completely removed, attention is turned toward the outer nucleus. But that's another chapter.

Conclusion

Spring surgery is a very controlled, straightforward way to remove a cataract. The sequence of the steps is logical, and the emphasis on sculpting and nuclear plate shaving makes the phaco tip do most of the work. This technique avoids a lot of nuclear manipulation, like repeated rotation, prolapse, or separation of nuclear segments with cracking of the posterior plate. It is almost a one-handed technique. The second instrument is used for a single 180° rotation and not much more. I recommend this method as a reasonably simple technique for converting from planned extracap directly to endocapsular phacoemulsification in cases involving pine-tree cataracts.

Making the Transition

The first thing you will probably have to do in making the transition to using the phaco machine is retrain your feet. When the right foot is dominant, the phaco control pedal will be placed on the right where the microscope control pedal is usually located. You will have to get used to the microscope pedal being on the left. (If your left foot is dominant, invert these instructions.)

You can make the transition to phaco in stages. First, practice handling instruments through a small incision by switching to automated I&A of cortex if you have not already been using it. Leave several ports of entry through the incision to the anterior chamber in early cases. This allows you to insert the probe at various angles and gain access to all of the cortex. In subsequent cases, suture the wound to leave only one entry point so you can get a feel for how the probe must be swivelled around inside the eye through a small incision.

The next stage, once the phaco machine arrives and the staff is thoroughly familiar with its operation, is to make your usual incision and can-opener capsulotomy, then sculpt the nucleus with the phaco probe a bit before doing your nucleus expression.

A partially sculpted nucleus cannot be handled like an unsculpted nucleus, however. For one thing, it is very unfriendly to the corneal endothelium. You probably have aspirated most of the viscoelastic in the anterior chamber while practicing sculpting. Before you convert to nucleus expression, you must re-instill viscoelastic to protect the endothelium.

After you feel comfortable with sculpting, try a relaxing nucleotomy before converting to your expression technique. Keep with this staged program until you're doing the whole spring procedure in all of your soft, pine-tree cataracts. For hard, oak-tree cataracts we'll need another technique.

Two Phaco Techniques

These illustrations summarize the techniques described in the chapters. There are really two techniques used, depending on the type of cataract: spring surgery for soft lenses and a four-quadrant nuclear cracking maneuver for hard ones. But both techniques start the same way.

Hydrodissection

Figure 1. The "hydro" maneuvers (Chapter 4) allow the hard inner nucleus to be rotated in the bag while the softer outer layers act as a cushion. Thorough hydrodissection is absolutely essential to both of our phaco techniques.

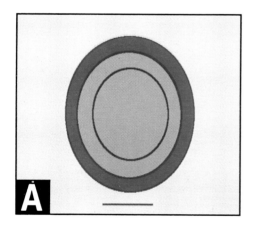

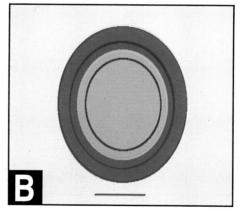

A. The gray cataract is shown behind the blue iris, with the crystalline lens held in place behind a capsulorhexis anterior capsulotomy.

B. Hydrodissection of the inner and outer nuclear layers will produce the well-known "golden ring." If this does not appear, hydrodelineation is not complete. There must be complete separation of the inner nucleus, not just a wash of fluid around the cortex and capsule.

Spring Surgery

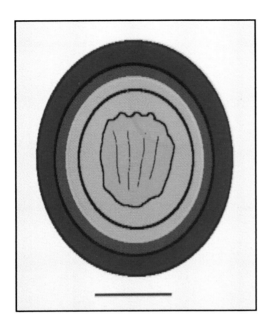

Sculpting

Figure 2. Sculpting (Chapter 5) is the easiest part of phaco. In the spring surgery technique for soft cataracts (Chapter 6), we want to sculpt out quite a bit of the nuclear core and leave fairly wide "handles" on either side of the sculpted area. These will be used a little later on. If we find that the cataract is very hard and inflexible, we will change to our four-quadrant cracking technique (Chapter 7).

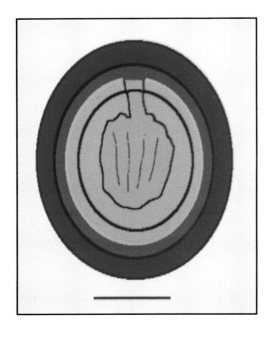

Relaxing nucleotomy

Figure 3. The relaxing nucleotomy maneuver (Chapters 5 and 6) is performed with the phaco probe held steady, port down, at the inferior nucleus. Pulsed phaco power will bring the nucleus up to the probe, creating a hole in the edge of the bowl left by sculpting.

Figure 4. The relaxing nucleotomy is enlarged. This destruction of the nuclear bowl is necessary to allow the folding maneuver that is used later in spring surgery.

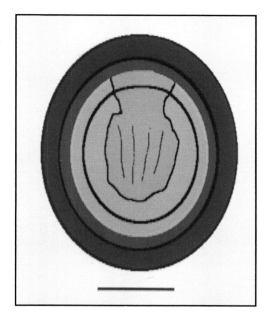

Figure 5. The nucleus is then rotated (**A**) to bring the relaxing nucleotomy around 180° (**B**).

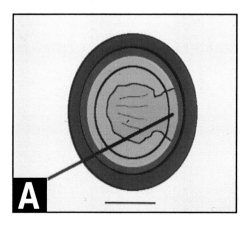 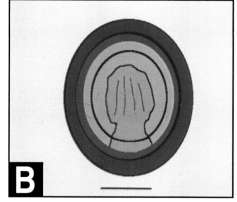

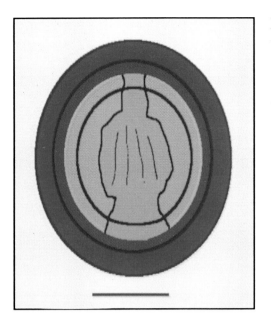

Figure 6. Another relaxing nucleotomy is made directly opposite the first.

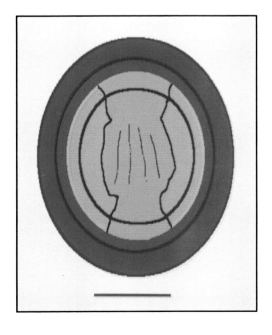

Figure 7. Again, enlargement of the nucleotomy prepares the nuclear handles.

Posterior plate shaving

Figure 8. Posterior plate shaving (Chapter 5) is maneuver that often inspires fear. It is not a blind maneuver, however, since the tip does not go under the iris. And so long as there is lens tissue visible, the capsule is safe. When you shave down an area to where the red reflex shows through, that serves as a guide for the thickness of the rest of the posterior plate.

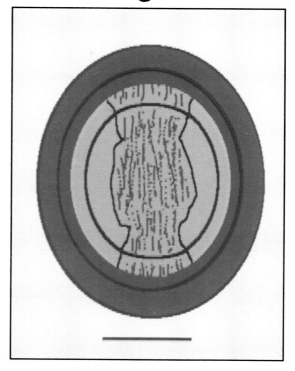

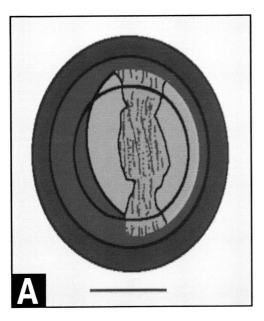

Folding the wings

Figure 9. The peripheral aspiration and removal maneuver (PAAR, as described in Chapter 5) is used to fold the two wings on the hinge of thin posterior nuclear plate.

A. One nuclear handle is aspirated and then drawn away from the capsular bag...

B. ...where it is emulsified and removed safely away from the capsule.

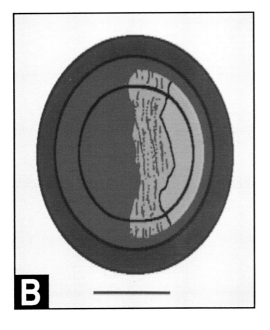

Figure 10. The PAAR maneuver is repeated in mirror image.

A. The other nuclear handle is aspirated and then drawn away from the capsular bag...

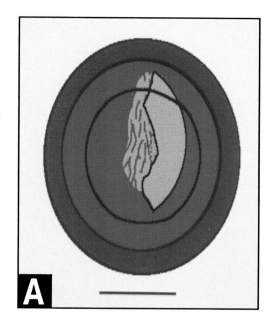

B. ...where it too is emulsified and removed.

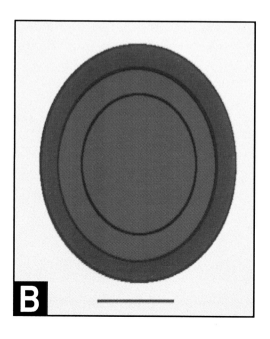

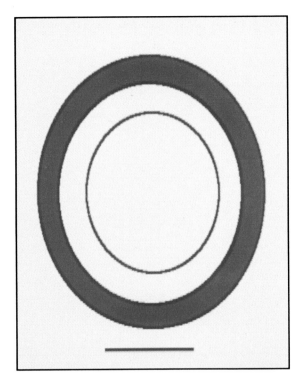

Figure 11. The outer nucleus is aspirated away from the capsular fornix, teased into the plane of the anterior capsule, and removed using gentle aspiration and emulsification (Chapter 8).

Four-Quadrant Cracking

Figure 12. The spring surgery technique is designed for the removal of soft, flexible cataracts. The folding maneuvers can only be carried out on a nucleus that will bend like the branches of a pine tree (Chapter 5). Some cataracts are hard and brittle, however, like oak trees. These are best removed with a cracking technique (Chapter 7).

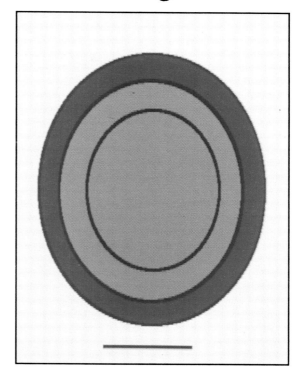

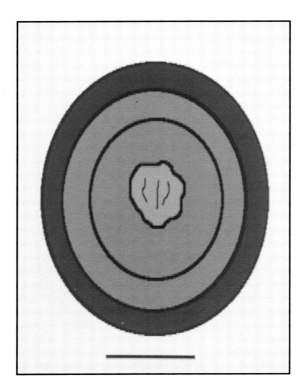

Sculpting

Figure 13. Sculpting is carried out to a lesser degree in hard cataracts than in spring surgery. The strategy here will be to dig a trench for nuclear cracking.

Trench digging

Figure 14. The first trench is dug out through the periphery of the nucleus. The trench should be about two phaco tips wide. It's hard to get very deep in this initial trench-digging.

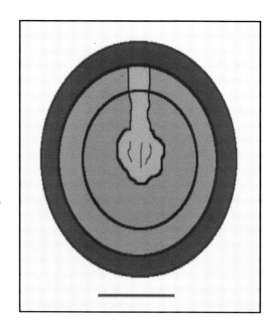

Figure 15. After the trench is completed, a spatula is inserted and the lens is rotated clockwise 90°

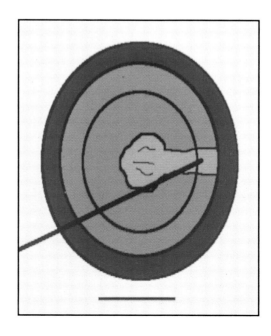

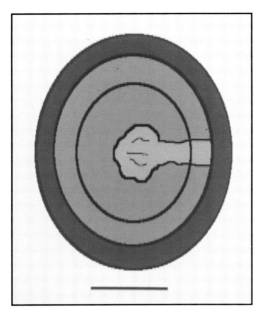

Figure 16. The trench-digging maneuvers will always be followed by *clockwise* rotation. This keeps each successive trench opposite the side port incision for easy manipulation with the spatula.

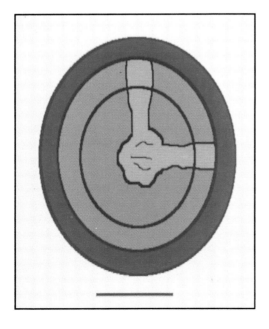

Figure 17. The trench-digging maneuver is repeated, beginning the separation of the nucleus into four quadrants.

Figure 18. After another clockwise 90° rotation, another trench is dug through the nucleus. Now that the first trench has been relocated just below the entry site of the phaco tip, the trench can be dug as deeply as necessary across the whole diameter of the nucleus.

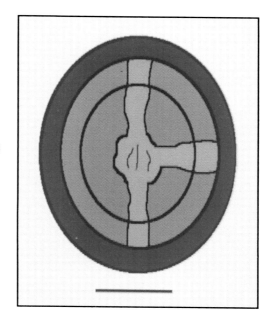

Figure 19. Another rotation and more trench-digging completes the division of the nucleus into quadrants for cracking.

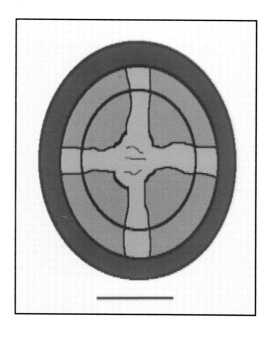

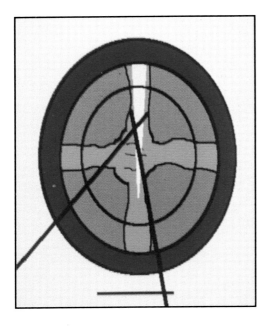

Cracking the posterior plate

Figure 20. Two instruments—in our technique, the phaco tip and a spatula—are used to crack the nucleus with a cross-instrument technique. The phaco tip presses against the left wall of the trench and the spatula presses against the right. The crack should split the nucleus down through the center of the lens.

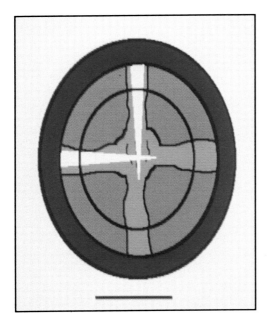

Figure 21. The lens is rotated—this time *counter*clockwise—and the cracking maneuver is repeated to completely isolate the first quadrant for emulsification.

Figure 22. By pressing the spatula against the anterior surface of the nucleus toward the 4:30 position, the apex of the quadrant (green area) will be elevated away from the posterior capsule. This is the point at which the nuclear quadrant is engaged with the phaco tip.

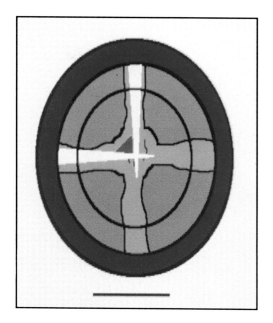

Figure 23. The nuclear quadrant is emulsified within the capsular bag, holding the spatula against the nuclear quadrant for stability.

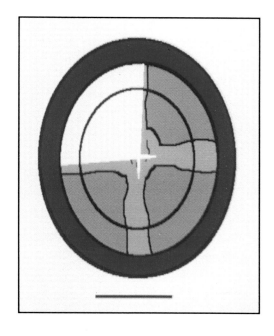

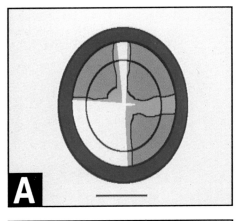

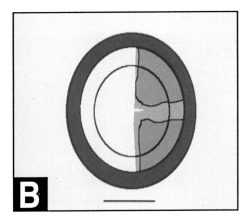

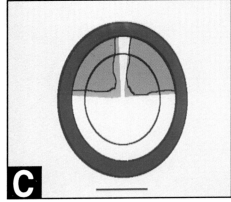

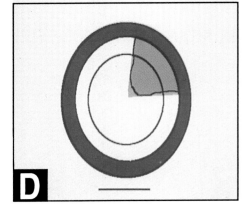

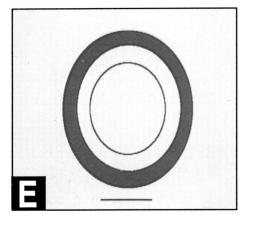

Emulsifying the quadrants

Figure 24. A. Counterclockwise rotation is necessary to bring the next trench into place for cracking. **B.** The same manipulations of the spatula and phaco tip are used to emulsify the next quadrant. **C.** Another rotation. **D.** Another quarter is emulsified. **E.** The final rotation and emulsification are performed. By this time the outer nucleus is usually gone. If not, it is removed as described in Chapter 8.

7

Four Quadrant Cracking

Howard Gimbel has to be considered the father of all the nuclear cracking operations. His divide-and-conquer technique is the prototype for all the operations that break cataracts into several small pieces for removal through the small capsulorhexis opening. The specific method of four quadrant cracking is a modification originally described by John Shepherd. For those cataracts which I characterize as being oak tree cataracts, I do not think that there is a better operation than four quadrant cracking. It is a very reasonable and rational operation in its application of physiologic forces to crack the posterior plate of the cataract.

Evaluating the cataract

I make my determination whether to proceed with spring surgery or four quadrant cracking during the first few sculpting passes. If I get the sensation that I can remove anywhere from half to one full tip width of tissue on each pass, I consider the cataract to be a soft one and I proceed with spring surgery. If, on the other hand, I try to sculpt and find that I can remove no more than a quarter to a half of a tip width with each pass, I change my strategy immediately to allow the four quadrant cracking operation to be performed.

Technique

Quartering the nucleus

It is still necessary to do some sculpting before four quadrant cracking, but it is not carried as wide as in spring surgery (Figure 13; we're looking again at the color drawings that appear in a separate section immediately before this chapter).

The strategy is to follow a moderate amount of sculpting with some trench digging to carve a narrow gully right down the middle of the cataract. The gully should be made as deep as possible and about two phaco tip widths wide (Figure 14). Later in the operation we are going to use the phaco tip and a second instrument to crack apart the posterior plate. A trench about two tip widths wide is sufficient to get both instruments in.

You will find that the first trench cannot be made very deep because uncut tissue in the subincisional area will prevent your phaco tip from getting down to clean out the bottom of the trench. Don't worry about it. In a few minutes you will have better access to this tissue.

After the first trench is made, insert your spatula through the side port and rotate the nucleus 90° clockwise (Figure 15). Make another trench in the inferior nucleus, beginning the process of quartering the cataract.

The clockwise direction of rotation is important. This is going to keep the trenches on the opposite side of the eye from the spatula entry point (Figure 16), so you will always have someplace to plant the spatula and control the nucleus. When we crack the nucleus we will be rotating the nucleus counterclockwise in order to keep the intact pieces on the opposite side of the eye from the spatula, again for ease of manipulation.

After the second trench is dug (Figure 17), rotate the nucleus clockwise another 90° and make your third trench (Figure 18). Now you can remove the tissue that was originally in the subincisional area. This will allow you to finish the first trench. Once you've made the third trench out to the periphery, clean out the tissue overlying the posterior plate in the center of the nucleus. You should take the trench from 12 o'clock all the way to 6 o'clock, as deep as you feel comfortable making it.

Rotate the nucleus 90° once more and then make the fourth trench (Figure 19). Take this opportunity to complete the second trench, cleaning out the bottom of the gully as deeply as possible. You have now isolated four quadrants of inner nucleus separated by a thin bridge of posterior nuclear plate. All that is left now to do is crack this plate apart and remove each of the sections.

Cracking the nucleus

Some people take out all their instruments at this point and go back into the eye with a specialized nucleus cracker. I have never used any of these instruments, so I cannot make any recommendation about choosing one. I am not sure that they are necessary at all, however, because it is fairly easy to crack the nucleus simply using a spatula and the phaco tip.

Place your phaco tip in the inferior trench and press it against the left-hand wall. Place your spatula through the side port incision and press against the right-hand side of the trench. Using just a cross action, separate the two walls (Figure 20). You will see the posterior plate crack very easily in front of your eyes. If it does not crack, be more vigorous. If it still does not crack, shave the posterior plate some more to make it thinner. You should always make a special effort to thin out the posterior plate centrally during trench digging, because that is the thickest part of the cataract.

When you make your first crack be sure that you see it separate right down to the crossroads in the middle of the cataract. Then stop and rotate the nucleus one-quarter turn counterclockwise. Place your instruments into the new trench that is now at the 6 o'clock position and do another separation (Figure 21). Watch the crack form along the floor of this furrow, making sure that the crack extends to the crossroads. When it does, one quarter of nucleus (the quarter sitting between 3 and 6 o'clock) will be completely isolated from the rest of the cataract.

Press your spatula gently against the anterior wall of the cataract and push it toward the 4:30 position. This lifts the posterior apex of the quadrant, the part located at the crossroads of the trenches, up away from the posterior capsule (Figure 22). It will be pointing directly at your phaco tip. Place the tip right up against this corner, then begin aspiration and emulsification. The piece of nucleus will come directly toward your phaco tip without the tendency to spin or tumble (Figure 23).

This is a point where a lot of people make the mistake of grabbing the nucleus and pulling it up into the anterior chamber. If you do this, you'll break your anterior capsulotomy and emulsify the firm nucleus right next to the cornea. You'll end up with results comparable to anterior chamber phacoemulsification rather than in-the-bag phaco-emulsification: swollen, edematous corneas and transient poor visual acuities. Keep the phaco tip down in the capsular bag and emulsify the quadrants within the bag. That's the whole point of everything we've been trying to do.

Once the first quarter of nucleus is gone, rotate the nucleus another 90° counterclockwise and crack the posterior plate in the trench that is now at the 6 o'clock position. This isolates a second quarter between 3 and 6 o'clock. Again, press gently on the nucleus to lift the apex off the posterior capsule, then remove it just the same way you removed the first quarter.

Once again you'll rotate what is left of the nucleus 90°. Here you sometimes run into trouble because when there are only two quadrants left they are less stable in the bag and have a tendency to rotate or tumble. It might be necessary to stabilize the nucleus with the phaco tip and spatula. Sometimes you even have to thin out the posterior plate a little bit more because the cracking maneuver can be difficult. But once a crack is made, you end up with two quarters that can each be removed easily. But again, take great care to hold the phaco tip down in the capsular bag and emulsify the nucleus there rather than pulling it out of the bag (Figure 24).

Discussion

Keep in mind that we are doing this operation on oak tree cataracts, the cataracts that have a natural physiologic tendency to crack easily. We are not using this technique on the soft pine tree cataracts. Those cataracts are frustrating to crack because physiologically they want to flex. That's why we take them out with the spring surgery technique. If you try to crack them, the posterior plate just stretches.

A word of caution. Sometimes the central area of the cataract is neglected during the trench-digging phase of the four quadrant cracking procedure. If this is the case, you will get a cataract that cracks beautifully in the periphery and mid-trench, but at the point where all four trenches meet the tissue refuses to separate because the plate is still too thick. Prevent this by being sure that it has been shaved adequately.

Four quadrant cracking is a very well-defined operation in which specific steps are performed sequentially. The keys to this technique are diligence and patience. It is done on a very firm nucleus, so everything takes a little bit longer than you might expect. When you get the hang of it, you might say that this operation looks as though it were choreographed. Each operation will be performed in exactly the same way. I think you will enjoy doing it.

8

Removing the Outer Nucleus

Whether you perform spring surgery or four quadrant cracking, there remains an outer nuclear shell that has to be removed. It is a reasonably simple task to put the phaco tip up against the shell at the 6 o'clock position and pull it toward you, teasing it away from the capsular bag. You might also use your spatula to help flip it over—the "flip" part of Howard Fine's chip-and-flip technique.

Sometimes, however, it is difficult to gain a purchase on the outer nucleus at 6 o'clock. You must then work to either side, rotating the phaco tip so that the bevel faces to the left or right to grasp a portion of the nucleus alongside the 6 o'clock position.

At other times you can grab the outer nucleus at 4 o'clock and sort of tease it in but, because the outer nucleus is so much larger than the capsulotomy opening, it does not flip over entirely. If that is the case, you can let go of the nucleus and rotate it a quarter turn, then grasp it again and pull. The outer nucleus frequently will roll up into something like a banana shape and then slip out through the capsulotomy. It usually is removed at the plane of the anterior capsule, using aspiration and emulsification as necessary.

It is always possible to aspirate a portion of the outer nucleus, bring it toward the capsulotomy and then emulsify it. This makes the nucleus smaller, but in general you should try to leave the outer nucleus intact so that it is easier to manipulate inside the eye up to the point when you're ready to aspirate the whole thing.

You don't have to worry about damaging the eye by flipping the outer nucleus over. This is a very soft structure and it molds itself to the shape of the capsular bag. Flipping over the outer nucleus is an entirely different activity than flipping over an inner nucleus. If you tumble an inner nucleus, you can do serious damage to the capsule or (even worse) the corneal endothelium. Tumbling and folding the outer nucleus, however, presents no such risk to the intraocular structures. And you will find that removing the outer nucleus becomes much easier.

9

Cortical Aspiration

Cortical aspiration in phacoemulsification is much different than cortical aspiration in extracapsular nucleus expression procedures. For one thing, there is much less cortex to remove. Some of it was washed away with the hydrodissection, and some of it came out with the outer nucleus. The closed system used in phacoemulsification also helps to maintain the depth of the capsular bag, and that makes it easier to get out the cortex. The continuous tear capsulotomy eliminates the capsular flaps that interfered with cortical aspiration through a can-opener capsulotomy, and that makes this step go easily.

Unfortunately, there is one big problem getting the cortex out after phacoemulsification in the bag with capsulorhexis, and that is the subincisional cortex. The anterior capsulotomy is small enough and the anterior capsule is large enough that you frequently have a hard time getting the phaco tip around to the subincisional area of the bag. We need a strategy for removing it.

Keep this in mind: if you can't get it... forget it.

Techniques

Side port cannulation

The first strategy for removing cortex from the subincisional area is to perform what I refer to as side port cannulation. This method uses a curved Simcoe cannula attached to a 3 cc syringe filled with BSS. Place the cannula through the side port incision and direct it under the anterior capsule where residual cortex remains (Figure 9-1). Press gently on the plunger of the syringe, and much of the cortex will be washed out into the middle of the capsular bag.

This is actually a type of enhanced hydrodissection. Once most of the cortex in the subincisional area has been irrigated, you can gently grasp some of it by pulling back on the plunger, thus generating a vacuum (Figure 9-2). Do not aspirate the cortex from the eye with the syringe. Tease it out of the capsular fornix. If you try to aspirate it, you will end up with a chamber collapse. Just get the cortex out of the fornix so you can go in with the I&A handpiece and remove all of it from the eye.

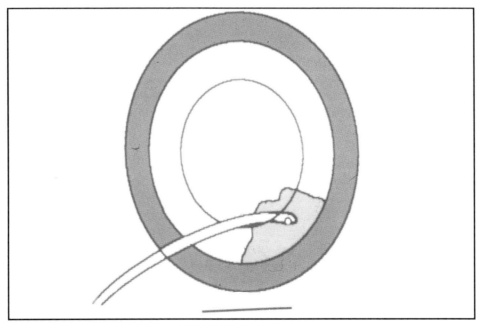

Figure 9-1. Side port cannulation is performed with a curved Simcoe cannula attached to a 3 cc syringe filled with BSS. The cannula is placed through the side port incision and directed under the anterior capsule where residual cortex remains. Gentle pressure on the plunger of the syringe washes much of the cortex out into the middle of the capsular bag.

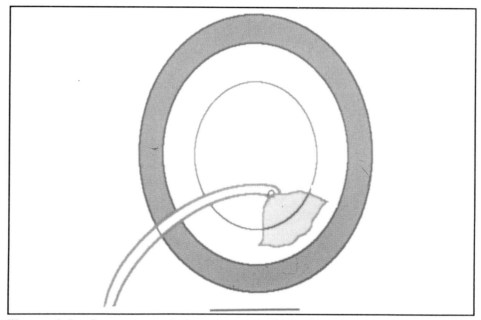

Figure 9-2. Once most of the cortex in the subincisional area has been irrigated, you can gently grasp it by pulling back on the plunger and generating a vacuum. Tease the cortex out of the capsular fornix rather than aspirating it from the eye. If you try to aspirate it, you will end up with a chamber collapse.

You might have to repeat these steps several times, but it is generally effective for getting out large amounts of subincisional cortex.

Viscoelastic technique

Another similar strategy is to put some viscoelastic in the eye, then go in and just aspirate out the cortex without irrigation. This technique wastes a lot of expensive viscoelastic and fails to loosen the cortex with irrigation. So unless you have a lot of viscoelastic lying around that you need to use up, as a rule you probably won't want to do this.

Of course there's an exception to the rule: the case where there is an opening in the posterior capsule. If there is a hole in the posterior capsule, you should definitely fill the eye with viscoelastic to hold the vitreous back and to open up the capsular bag (Figure 9-3). Then use your Simcoe cannula to aspirate the cortex gently from the capsular fornix as described above. Tease it away from its attachments, pull it

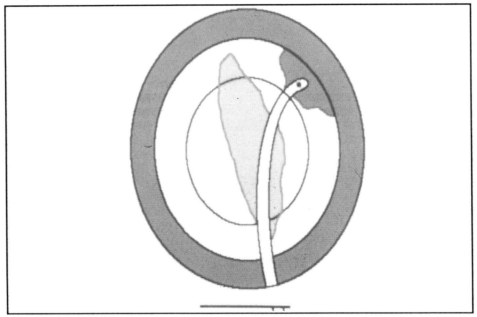

Figure 9-3. If there is a hole in the posterior capsule, fill the eye with viscoelastic before beginning cortical aspiration. This will hold the vitreous back and open up the capsular bag.

all the way out of the incision and irrigate it away after it is out of the eye (Figure 9-4). If you do this, you can get out almost all of the cortex without ever disturbing the vitreous. Simply replenish the viscoelastic every so often as necessary to keep everything in place. (The next chapter is all about vitrectomy, and I'll be elaborating on this type of viscoelastic technique there.)

Other strategies

Those are my preferred methods for removing the subincisional cortex. Let's take a look at a few others that I have tried and you may find useful some day.

One method is to use a U-shaped cannula through the phaco incision. You have to insert the cannula into the incision sideways, rotate it until the opening is under the anterior capsule, then squirt and aspirate. These cannulas work very well, but I find it easier to aspirate the subincisional cortex using a Simcoe cannula through the side port.

Another way to remove the subincisional cortex is by a method

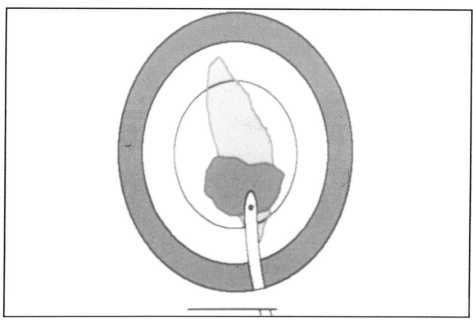

Figure 9-4. Aspirate the cortex gently from the capsular fornix with the Simcoe cannula, tease it away from its attachments, pull it out of the incision and irrigate it away after it is out of the eye. Replenish the viscoelastic as necessary.

that I call capsular retraction. In this technique you first widen the incision to the width necessary for intraocular lens implantation (anywhere from 5 to 6 mm) and then go through that incision with two instruments: a Kuglen hook, which retracts the iris and the anterior capsule, and the I&A tip, which performs the cortical aspiration. This is a bit of an awkward maneuver unless there is a lot of cortex there. I generally do not do it much anymore.

    Another technique that also works very well, especially if there is a lot of cortex left, is to open up the incision, put the intraocular lens in the capsular bag and then rotate the lens about 180°. The haptics sweeping through the capsular fornix during rotation will wipe out the cortex, allowing it to float away from the fornix where it can be easily aspirated with the I&A handpiece.

10

Vitrectomy Techniques

The concept of vitreous loss during phacoemulsification requires some consideration, because the vitreous acts differently here than it does in nucleus expression procedures. The closed system of phaco-emulsification has certain advantages in limiting the damage caused by vitreous loss and in enhancing the surgeon's ability to perform an appropriate vitrectomy (Figure 10-1).

If vitreous loss occurs in a nucleus expression procedure, there are no natural forces to limit the flow of vitreous out of the eye (Figure 10-2). Vitreous loss is directly related to the size of the incision and to the liquidity of the vitreous gel. In phacoemulsification, on the other hand, the constant pressure in the anterior chamber helps to hold the vitreous back, and the small incision limits how much vitreous can extrude from the eye.

The pressure in the anterior chamber in such a closed system can even prevent vitreous loss. If the posterior capsule is opened during the operation, but the vitreous face remains intact, the anterior chamber pressure can hold the vitreous back and prevent vitreous loss. Even if the vitreous face is disturbed and vitreous is prepared to move forward, the pressure in the anterior chamber can still hold it back, preventing loss or at least limiting the vitreous movement to a mild prolapse into the anterior chamber.

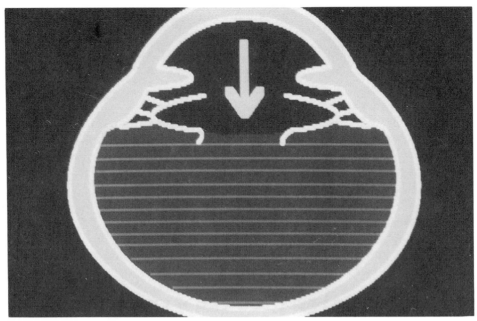

Figure 10-1. Vitreous loss in phacoemulsification can be limited because the procedure maintains a closed system. Anterior chamber pressure (arrow) will press against the vitreous and hold it back.

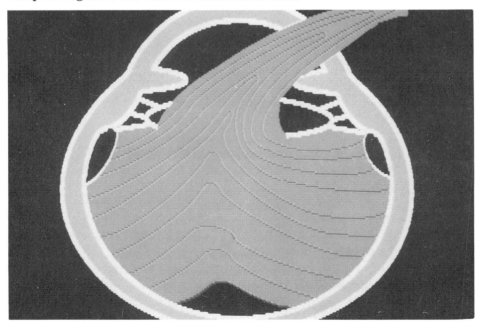

Figure 10-2. In procedures without a closed system, such as nucleus expression and intracapsular cataract extraction, the vitreous is not contained. The amount lost can be significant, exerting tension on the vitreous base and vitreomacular interface.

True vitreous loss can occur if the posterior capsule opens suddenly, or if it opens in such a way that you don't recognize it immediately: if it's behind a piece of nucleus, for example. The aspiration port of the phaco handpiece will remove fluid from the anterior chamber, and the fluid will be replaced partially by solution from the irrigation bottle and partially by vitreous. Further aspiration may result in vitreous being aspirated to the phaco tip with further loss. In a sense, the amount of vitreous loss is directly related to the time between the opening of the posterior capsule and the moment when the surgeon recognizes it.

Analogy of the Slinky

This discussion of vitreous loss and vitrectomy techniques revolves around an analogy involving a Slinky toy. You may remember this toy—it's been around for several decades. It is a floppy spring that can be used in a variety of playful ways. It comes in a variety of sizes and colors, just as the vitreous comes with many individual characteristics, but for now, let's consider the Slinky as representing an "average" vitreous.

One good example of how the vitreous acts like a Slinky occurs in the vitreous wick syndrome. A small, narrow band of vitreous is stretched to the incision. Tension is placed right on through the vitreous body, disturbing the retina, and cystoid macular edema develops. Severing the vitreous band near the incision causes the rest of it to retract quickly in the eye, like the retraction of a spring. The cystoid macular edema often will resolve.

Another example is a Weck-Cel vitrectomy. With the Weck-Cel, some vitreous can be pulled out of the eye to be cut. The "lost" vitreous retracts quickly into the eye.

We will consider the study of vitreous dynamics by imagining it as a tiny Slinky. We will imagine that a Slinky is attached to the vitreous base and another attached to the vitreomacular interface. If the Slinky is pulled just a little bit, the forces will be absorbed by the first few coils of the spring and not much will happen (Figure 10-3). If it is pulled a lot, the entire coil will stretch out and exert tension at its base (Figure 10-4). In the case of our imaginary vitreous Slinkies, that would put tension on the vitreous base, leading to a detached retina, and on the vitreomacular interface, leading to cystoid macular edema.

This leads us to the first principle of vitrectomy.

Do not stretch the Slinky. The best way to avoid stretching the Slinky is to maintain an intact posterior capsule. If that is not

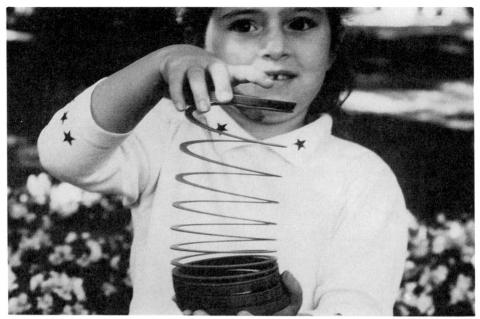

Figure 10-3. The vitreous can be compared with a Slinky toy. Gentle stretching disturbs only the first few coils of the toy, leaving the main body undisturbed.

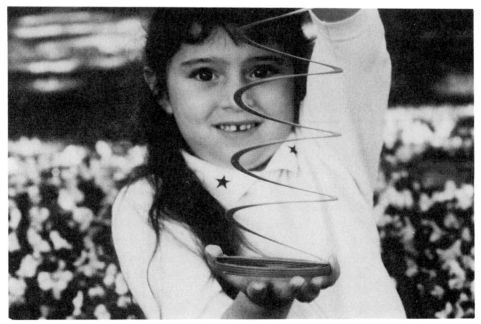

Figure 10-4. If there is a lot of tension on the Slinky, all of the coils are disturbed and the tension is transmitted right down to its base—likewise with the vitreous body.

possible, we have to maintain as much of the integrity of the vitreous as possible by spotting the tear and stopping the aspiration. This may prevent all vitreous loss. If vitreous moves into the anterior chamber, however, a vitrectomy will be necessary.

If the vitrectomy is performed with a coaxial infusion cannula slipped over the vitrectomy tip (Figure 10-5), a one-handed vitrectomy is possible but disturbs the Slinky in three separate ways.

1. Extension of the posterior capsular tear. The force of the infusion is in the same direction as the tip is pointing. That means the infusion will be directed downward into the deep areas of the eye. As the tip passes down toward an opening in the posterior capsule, the infusion flow will strike the capsular flaps and force them apart. This extends the capsular tear and enlarges the opening, The result is more vitreous prolapsing forward and stretching the Slinky (Figure 10-6).

   Traditionally, we have considered the posterior capsule as the only structural barrier to vitreous movement, but the anterior capsule is also a barrier. This is especially true with a small capsulorhexis. Trying to get vitreous to prolapse through a 4.5-mm capsulorhexis is like trying to squeeze toothpaste through the top of the tube. The small, rigid opening limits how much you can stretch the Slinky. This may turn out to be one of the most significant benefits of the capsulorhexis capsulotomy.

2. Hydration of the vitreous. The infusion fluid hydrates the vitreous, increasing its volume and causing it to expand. The only direction the vitreous is able to expand is toward the anterior chamber through the opening in the posterior capsule. This forward motion stretches the Slinky (Figure 10-7).

3. Flushing the vitreous. The force of the infusion acts like a high-pressure hose and pushes the vitreous around, shaking and wiggling it, forcing the Slinky every which way and exerting trauma to the Slinky's bases (the vitreous base and the vitreomacular interface). The vitreous is moving even in low flow systems, creating microtraumas. The result of all this movement is that the vitreous is flushed out of the back of the eye toward the anterior chamber (Figure 10-8). This pulls the body toward the anterior chamber, increasing the amount of vitreous that needs to be removed. This is what happens when what looks like a small vitrectomy turns into a large one. The anterior chamber is constantly refilled with new vitreous until a significant amount of it has been removed (Figure 10-9).

Each of these three forces adversely affects the integrity of the vitreous because each of them causes the Slinky to stretch, exerting more force at the Slinky's base. It is not surprising that vitrectomy

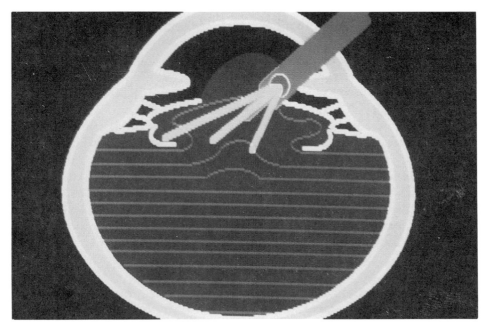

Figure 10-5. Vitrectomy tip with a coaxial cannula in place. Don't do this.

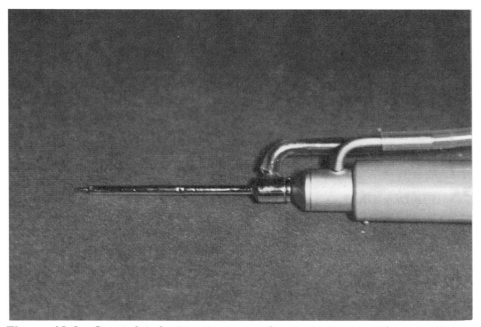

Figure 10-6. Coaxial infusion rips open the posterior capsule, permitting more vitreous to prolapse, stretching the Slinky.

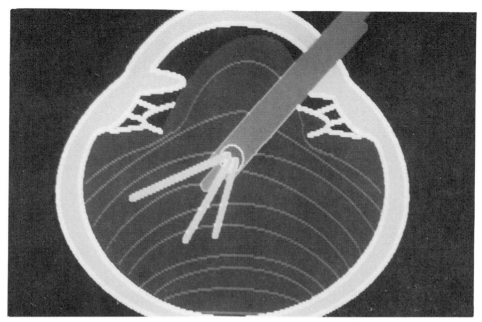

Figure 10-7. Coaxial infusion also hydrates the vitreous, forcing more of it into the anterior chamber and again stretching the Slinky.

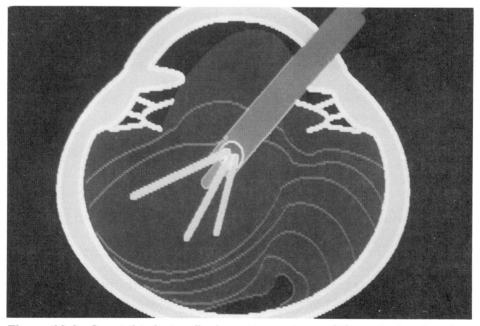

Figure 10-8. Coaxial infusion flushes vitreous toward the anterior chamber, stretching and wiggling the Slinky.

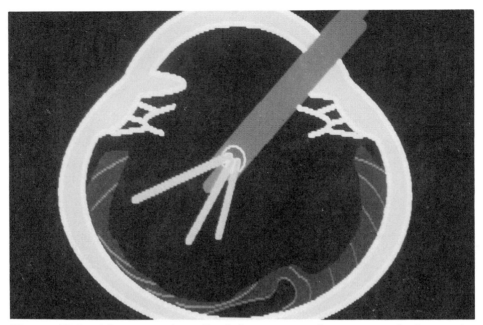

Figure 10-9. After removing all of the vitreous that was washed into the anterior chamber, a lot of the vitreous cavity has been disturbed, including the vitreomacular interface and the vitreous base.

following vitreous loss in cataract surgery has a postoperative complication rate of 30% to 50%.

The best strategy in performing a vitrectomy is to touch the vitreous as little as possible. With the closed system of phaco, there is a limit to how much the vitreous can move on its own. The key is to avoid violating any more of the vitreous. If you can remove the vitreous from the anterior chamber without disturbing the rest of the vitreous, especially that overlying the vitreous base of the vitreomacular interface, you should have very few postoperative problems. This can be accomplished by adhering to the second principle of vitrectomy.

Use a bimanual technique with a separate infusion line. To avoid the problems caused by coaxial infusion, remove the coaxial sleeve and replace it with a separate infusion line (Figure 10-10). A chamber maintainer is a short piece of silicone tubing with a female Leur-lock connector on one end and a short hub on the other. Connect the Leur-lock connector to the infusion line from the vitrectomy infusion bottle. The tubing can be held in the left hand and the hub placed into the side port incision when needed.

The vitrectomy tip is held in the right hand and passed into the

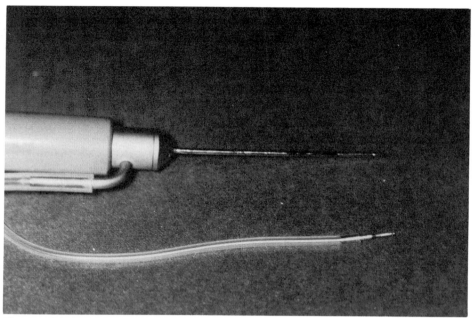

Figure 10-10. Bimanual vitrectomy is performed with the infusion separated from the cutting tip. The separate infusion line is attached to the infusion port of the vitrectomy unit and aspiration is connected to the cutting tip.

eye, down through the vitreous in the anterior chamber, through the opening in the posterior capsule, and held a millimeter or two behind the posterior capsule. The aspiration port is directed upward toward the cornea (Figure 10-11).

The strategy is to draw the vitreous in the anterior chamber down to the vitrectomy tip until no more vitreous is in the anterior chamber, then stop (Figure 10-12). We specifically do not want to remove any more vitreous from the vitreous cavity other than cleaning up around the posterior capsule. The body of the vitreous should remain unviolated so we will not disturb the Slinky further. Which is our third principle of vitrectomy.

It is unfortunate if the Slinky is stretched due to vitreous loss, but it is worse if the surgeon stretches it any more. After the vitrectomy tip is in position just behind the posterior capsule, gentle cutting and aspiration can be activated to draw the vitreous down from the anterior chamber to the vitrectomy tip. This does not disturb the rest of the vitreous, but it does soften the eye. After awhile, the eye needs to be firmed up again and irrigation is required.

The irrigation line is placed into the side port incision, and the flow of the fluid is directed across the anterior chamber in the plane

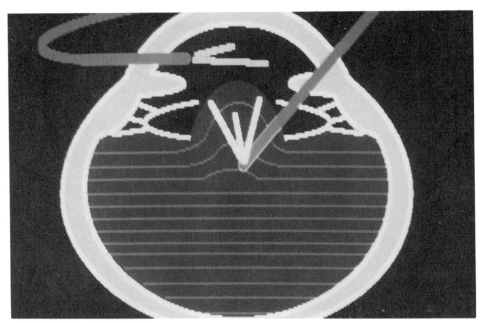

Figure 10-11. The infusion is directed parallel to the iris. The cutting tip is placed behind the posterior capsule and the vitreous in the anterior chamber is aspirated downward. The body of the vitreous is not disturbed.

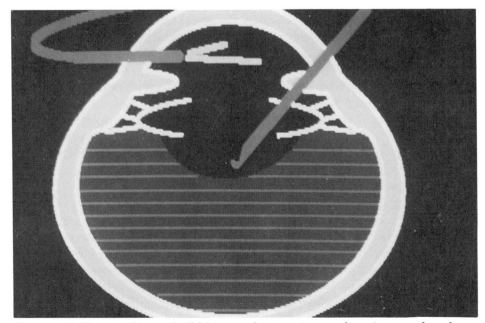

Figure 10-12. At the end of bimanual vitrectomy, the vitreous has been removed from the anterior chamber, the capsular bag, and the region just behind the posterior capsule. The rest of the vitreous has not been touched.

of the iris. The goal is to refill the anterior chamber without pushing any of the irrigation fluid behind the posterior capsule. Some admixing of the fluid and the vitreous in the anterior chamber may occur, but that is not important. It I will all be removed anyway. The important thing is not to mix irrigation fluid with the vitreous behind the posterior capsule, because that hydration will lead to new vitreous prolapse. This forms the basis for the fourth principle of vitrectomy.

The infusion maintains the anterior chamber; it has no role in the vitreous cavity. When the vitrectomy has proceeded to the point where the vitreous is out of the anterior chamber, a little more has to be done near the posterior chamber to eliminate any traction or adhesions. Then you are finished. The posterior capsule is usually unaffected by the vitrectomy, and insertion of a posterior chamber intraocular lens can be performed without difficulty, although it usually must be placed in the ciliary sulcus rather than in the capsular bag. But this depends on the size of the opening in the posterior capsule.

If residual cortex is in the capsular bag, it can be removed with the vitrectomy tip using a combination of aspiration and cutting. Because aspiration of the cortex sometimes leads to new vitreous prolapse, the cutter will have to be activated at the first sign of aspiration blockage to sever the vitreous before any tension is exerted.

Another method of cortical aspiration is to hold the vitreous back with a viscoelastic and remove the cortex with a manual aspirator, such as a cannula on a syringe. If the anterior chamber shallows during cortical aspiration, it has to be refilled with viscoelastic to maintain a positive pressure against the vitreous.

Results

I reviewed our results in 3,300 consecutive cases of phacoemulsification with lens implantation (Table 10-1). The posterior capsule was inadvertently opened in 102 cases (3.0%), but vitreous loss occurred in only 32 cases (1%). And in only two of these cases did cystoid macula edema develop. I think these results can be attributed to the unique advantages of the closed system of phacoemulsification and to the fact that aspiration was terminated before vitreous was aspirated.

All of the patients with vitreous loss were treated exactly as described in this chapter. Two of them (6%) developed CME, in each case with permanent vision loss: one to 20/40 and the other to 20/200. The rest (94%) had what I considered to be a normal postoperative

Total cases	3,300	
Nature of complication	No.	%
Posterior capsule openings	102	3%
Vitreous loss	32	1%
Posterior capsule openings resulting in vitreous loss	33%	
Timing of vitreous loss	No.	% (of 32)
At end of cortical aspiration	8	25%
During emulsification	11	34%
At end of emulsification	13	41%

Table 10-1. Vitrectomy during phacoemulsification.

course, with recovery of corrected vision to 20/20 by the third postoperative week. All of these patients were followed for more than a year, during which time they all maintained 20/20 vision. I believe that this study's low incidence of CME (6% compared with the usually reported level of 30% to 50%) is a result of adhering to the principles described in this chapter.

Bimanual vitrectomy is a gentler and safer way to perform vitrectomy after vitreous loss during phacoemulsification because it does not stretch the Slinky. By following the principles presented, it is possible to limit the morbidity and enhance visual acuity in eyes with vitreous loss as in those without vitreous loss.

11

Viscoelastic Materials

Three viscoelastics dominate the market: Healon (sodium hyaluronate, Pharmacia), Viscoat (hyaluronic acid and chondroitin sulfate, Alcon) and Occucoat (hydroxypropylmethylcellulose, Storz Ophthalmics). They are different materials with different properties. In some procedures, they are not interchangeable.

Pseudoplasticity

We are used to Newtonian fluids like water or air, where the viscosity of the fluid is independent of the shear rate (that is, how quickly an object is moving through it). Chondroitin sulfate is a Newtonian fluid. Other viscoelastic materials are non-Newtonian fluids, where viscosity decreases with increasing shear rate. A stationary object in a non-Newtonian fluid is wrapped in an area of higher viscosity than is a moving object. This is sometimes referred to as the pseudoplasticity of viscoelastics, and all three major brands exhibit the property to some degree.

Healon has a much greater pseudoplasticity than Viscoat or Occucoat. At shear rates near zero, it is a very viscous material—more viscous than either of the other two. At high shear rates, it is much less viscous than the others. In practical terms, this means that

Healon is excellent for maintaining the anterior chamber as well as for letting instruments pass freely.

Elasticity

The elasticity of a viscoelastic (the tendency to return to normal shape after being extended) is generally measured as viscosity at a shear rate of 0. Healon is thus also the most elastic of our viscomaterials.

During IOL insertion, the viscosity of the viscoelastic is what helps protect the endothelium against compressive forces, but it also transmits the drag force on the lens. Since viscosity is also temperature dependent, chilled infusion will enhance the transmission of drag forces to the endothelium. High pseudoplasticity will help compensate for these tendencies, so we find Healon advantageous during IOL insertion.

Cohesion

Cohesion (often called followability) is an important characteristic when it is time to remove the material. Healon comes out of the eye easily, in one "blob," because it is cohesive. Viscoat has low cohesion and thus cannot be removed as easily. Occucoat has greater cohesion, but not as much as Healon.

What does this mean for our phaco technique? A highly cohesive material will tend to come out of the eye quickly as soon as you start emulsifying and aspirating the nucleus. Healon will form the anterior chamber well because of its high viscosity, but its high cohesion also means that it will be sucked out of the eye with the high flow of phacoemulsification. Viscoat and Occucoat offer advantages in that regard. Pharmacia is introducing Healon GV, a less cohesive formulation, to maintain the anterior chamber better during phaco.

Contact angle is often discussed in relation to IOL materials, but also bears upon viscoelastic behavior. A lower contact angle, indicating hydrophilicity, will mean better coating of the corneal endothelium. Occucoat has the lowest contact angle of the three materials. Significantly, it is promoted as a viscoadherent. Viscoat has a higher contact angle than Occucoat, but not as high as Healon.

In general, for low-flow, low-turbulence tissue manipulation procedures such as ECCE, a viscomaterial with the highest viscosity at shear rate 0 (Healon) is most suitable. For high-flow, high-turbulence procedures, low contact angle and low cohesion are more suitable. Viscoat and Occucoat are preferable in phacoemulsification. I have not used Orcolon (polyacrilamide, Optical Radiation Corp.), which has physical characteristics quite similar to hyaluronic acid. A viscoelastic derived from human placenta (Collagel, Domilens) is available in France. This material has a pseudoplasticity even greater than Healon. I have not used either of these materials personally, however, so I cannot comment on their relative merits.

12

Conclusion: Making Your Transition

That's it. That's how I do it and I think that's how you can do it too. All the steps are reasonably logical and, at least to me, they make sense. There is nothing magically difficult about this operation. It just requires a little bit of planning to work out a strategy and then you can proceed safely.

If you are already performing phacoemulsification, you can pick up a number of the steps presented in this book very easily. You can modify your incision one time and then modify a capsulotomy another time but, once you modify your capsulotomy to the continuous tear capsulotomy, you are obligated to perform in the bag phacoemulsification and not iris plane phacoemulsification.

If you are not performing phacoemulsification already, there are a few positive steps you can take toward performing the procedure.

The first thing I would do is take one of the established phacoemulsification courses. There are a few that have been around for quite a while and I want you to specifically ask your friends and look out for a course that is positive in tone. Look for a course that actually encourages you to perform the operation and try to avoid one which tries to make the operation seem harder than it is.

Sometimes you cannot find out what a course is like until you take it, but if you ask around you can get some feeling for what courses are out there.

The next thing I would do is use your machine manufacturer's representative as a resource. All of them can arrange practice sessions using plastic or animal eyes to help you familiarize yourself with the use of the machine and using it in a clinical setting.

The next thing I would do is make small modifications in your extracapsular technique. For example, you can make the phacoemulsification incision and then stop and turn it into your standard extracapsular incision and then continue your operation the same way as always.

Another thing you can do is a continuous tear capsulotomy but then when you are done do a can opener capsulotomy outside that or at least put a series of relaxing incisions in the anterior capsule before trying to express the nucleus. Remember that it is not wise to routinely try to express the nucleus through a continuous tear capsulotomy. There are methods which will permit you to do that but for purposes of this discussion it is not a good idea.

The next thing you can practice is hydrodissection and the other hydro step. In fact, I will encourage this because it will make your extracapsular procedures easier.

You can practice cortical aspiration using only one location on the limbus for access to the eye. This will simulate as much as possible performing cortical aspiration or, for that matter, phacoemulsification through a single port of entry.

If you have a phacoemulsification machine handy but you do not feel you are ready to perform the whole operation yet, you can do the steps just as I described above but also take the time to do some sculpting prior to expression of the nucleus. This will give you some practice with the tip inside the eye and boost your confidence because sculpting is a reasonably easy step.

And finally, when the day is right and all the parts come together, go ahead and do an entire phacoemulsification procedure and then another one and another one and never look back. You can do it because it is doable. If you can perform extracapsular surgery, you can perform phacoemulsification. The dexterity skills are the same. All you have to do is set your mind to it.

Good luck.

References
and Bibliography

References

Armeniades CD, Boriek A, Knolle GE: Effect of incision length, location, and shape on local corneoscleral deformation during cataract surgery. J Cataract Refract Surg 1990, 16(1):83-87.

Assia EI, Apple DJ, Barden A et al: An experimental study comparing various anterior capsulotomy technique. Arch Ophthalmol 1991, 109(5):642-647.

Koch DD: Presentation at Symposium on Cataract, IOL and Refractive Surgery, Los Angeles, March 1990.

Masket S: Keratorefractive aspects of the scleral pocket incision and closure method for cataract surgery. J Cataract Refract Surg 1989, 15(1)70-77.

Masket S: Deep versus appositional suturing of the scleral pocket incision for astigmatic control in cataract surgery. J Cataract Refract Surg 1987, 13(2) :13 1-13 5.

Pallin SL: Chevron incision for cataract surgery. J Cataract Refract Surg 1990, 16(6):779-781.

Russel TJ: Presentation at Symposium on Cataract, IOL and Refractive Surgery, Boston, April 1991.

Samuelson SW, Koch DD, Kuglen, CC: Determination of maximal incision length for true small-incision surgery. Ophthalmic Surg 1991, 22(4):204-207.

Sheperd JR: Induced astigmatism in small incision cataract surgery. J Cataract Refract Surg 1989, 15(1)85-88.

Singer, JA: Presentation at Symposium on Cataract, IOL and Refractive Surgery, Los Angeles, March 1990.

Bibliography

Apple DJ, Mamalis N, Olson RJ, Kincaid MC: Intraocular Lenses: Evolution, Designs, Complications and Pathology. Baltimore, Williams and Wilkins, 1989.

Devine TM, Banko W: Phacoemulsification Surgery. New York, Pergammon Press, 1991.

Gills JP, Sanders DR, eds: Small-incision Cataract Surgery. Thorofare, N.J., Slack, 1990, pp. 147-150.

Koch PS, Davison JA: Textbook of Advanced Phacoemulsification Techniques. Thorofare, N.J., Slack, 1990.

Kratz RP, Shammas HJ: Cataracts: Color Atlas of Ophthalmic Surgery. Philadelphia, J.B. Lippincott, 1991.

Maloney WF, Grindle L: Textbook of Phacoemulsification. Fallbrook, Calif., Lasenda Publishers, 1988.

Index